OXFORD MEDICAL PUBLICATIONS

Parkinson's Disease

THE FACTS

on or before the last date ...

PARKINSON'S DISEASE

THE FACTS

New Edition

GERALD STERN

*Consultant Neurologist, The Middlesex & University
College Hospitals; Honorary Consultant Neurologist,
The National Hospitals for Nervous Diseases, London*

and

ANDREW LEES

*Consultant Neurologist, The National Hospitals
for Nervous Diseases; The Middlesex & University
College Hospitals, London*

OXFORD   NEW YORK   TORONTO
OXFORD UNIVERSITY PRESS

Oxford University Press, Walton Street, Oxford OX2 6DP

London New York Toronto
Delhi Bombay Calcutta Madras Karachi
Kuala Lumpur Singapore Hong Kong Tokyo
Nairobi Dar es Salaam Cape Town
Melbourne Auckland Madrid
and associate companies in
Berlin Ibadan

Oxford is a trade mark of Oxford University Press

Published in the United States
by Oxford University Press Inc., New York

First published 1990
Reprinted 1991, 1993

British Library Cataloguing in Publication Data
Stern, Gerald
Parkinson's disease.—(Oxford medical publications)
1. Parkinson's disease
I. Title   II. Lees, Andrew
616.8'33   RC382
ISBN 0–19–261938–1
ISBN 0–19–261937–3 (pbk)

Library of Congress Cataloging in Publication Data
Stern, Gerald Malcolm
Parkinson's disease.
(Oxford medical publications)
Includes index.
I. Parkinsonism.   I. Lees, Andrew, 1947–
II. Title. {DNLM: 1. Parkinson's disease—Popular
works. WL 359 S839p}
RC382.S73   616.8'33   81–22485
ISBN 0–19–261938–1
ISBN 0–19–261937–3 (pbk)

Printed and bound in Great Britain by
Biddles Ltd, Guildford and King's Lynn

Foreword

E. J. P. Elliott
Chairman, Parkinson's Disease Society of the United Kingdom

I am delighted to be asked to write the foreword to the second edition of *Parkinson's Disease: The Facts*.

Since the first edition of this excellent book was published, the Parkinson's Disease Society has increased in size and strength. The Society is now in touch with over 40 000 patients, carers, and supporters, and has established some 148 branches in the United Kingdom. Its resources continue to be used in both the welfare of patients and in research. I am sure that *Parkinson's Disease: The Facts* will help all who come into contact with this condition.

Acknowledgements

Plates I and II by kind permission of Dr R. O. Barnard. We wish to thank Dr W. Olanow for Plate VIII and Dr R. Frackowiack for Plate IX.

Preface to the Second Edition

After an interlude of eight years our initial reasons for writing a book of this kind seem to be just as persuasive. It seems curious to recall that in the past many doctors were reluctant to mention frankly the diagnosis of Parkinson's disease. Even when the illness was of long-standing and obvious to relatives and friends—and, of course, to the patient too—frank and open discussion was avoided. It probably appeared kinder to enter a diplomatic conspiracy of silence with the family than to talk about a malady of unknown cause for which, at that time, there was little effective treatment available. While benevolently intended, such an approach often provoked needless fear and worry. It was common to hear how furtive consultations of aged textbooks and medical encyclopaediae led to grossly inaccurate notions about the illness.

Fortunately, in recent years we have witnessed radical changes. These include significant advances in our understanding of the malady and its treatment and, equally important, more sympathetic and understanding attitudes to disease and disability coupled with a warmer and more relaxed relationship between patient and doctor. Most people now expect open and informed discussion of their illness and if necessary are prepared to circumvent unduly anxious and over-protective relatives. While outdated library books have been replaced by vivid media presentations, these too may be over-dramatized, misunderstood, and potentially frightening. We share our patients' conviction that it is better to try and cope with known problems than unknown irrational fears. Accordingly, we attempted to write a reasonably accurate and comprehensible account of what was known and as yet unknown about Parkinson's disease couched in non-technical language. We were conscious that a book which attempts to give a brief overall description of a multi-faceted disease could never be an effective substitute for discussion of individual problems. This remains the sole province of a medical consultation.

In 1982, we attempted to answer six questions which, in our experience, patients and their families frequently asked about Parkinson's disease. We have been encouraged by the response and are very grateful for many useful comments and suggestions that we received. During the past eight years there have been several important developments and we now feel it timely to update some of our remarks. It is not yet possible to give complete answers, but we have tried to set out the known 'facts'. While the cause of the illness remains an enigma we have increasingly effective treatments for many symptoms and there are strong grounds for optimism about future developments. We hope that benefit and comfort will be gained from greater understanding of this common malady.

London   G.M.S.
September 1989   A.J.L.

Contents

1. What is Parkinson's disease?   1
2. What are the symptoms and course of Parkinson's
   disease?   13
3. What is the cause of Parkinson's disease?   21
4. What is the treatment?   31
5. How to live with Parkinson's disease   52
6. The future   60

Appendix I: Some useful addresses and contacts   66
Appendix II: Some helpful publications   77
Glossary   79
Index   83

Plates fall between pp. 22 and 23

1. What is Parkinson's disease?

In 1817, James Parkinson, an English physician, wrote a short essay describing six patients with a slowly progressive physical disease. He wrote that the illness was characterized by 'involuntary tremulous motion, with lessened muscular power, in parts not in action even when supported, with a propensity to bend the trunk forward and to pass from a walking to a running pace'. Throughout the world this illness is now called Parkinson's disease. The salient features are involuntary shaking movements of the limbs (tremor), stiffness of the muscles (rigidity), and slowness and poverty of movement (bradykinesia); from this triad of fundamental signs stem a wide variety of disabilities recognizable as changes in appearance, posture, and walking. The range and diversity of these symptoms will be discussed in greater detail, but it is important to emphasize that no patient closely resembles another and that each has unique problems.

James Parkinson

Patients and their families are usually very curious about James Parkinson and his achievements. He was born in 1755, the son of an apothecary and surgeon, spent his life in Shoreditch, then a village close to London, and died there at the age of 69. There is no known portrait of this remarkable man but he was described by a friend as 'rather below middle stature with an energetic, intelligent and pleasing countenance and of mild and courteous manner'. He was a passionate, outspoken man of many interests who enjoyed controversy and who was prepared to express his opinion on political, social, and scientific as well as medical matters. As a young man he was an ardent advocate of political reform and was responsible for a series of polemic pamphlets critical of the authorities of his time. He later turned his considerable energies to chemistry, geology, and palaeontology, and yet still found time to write prolifically on many medical matters. We would like to think that he would have approved of the aims of this book, because he wrote a primer of medicine for the lay reader entitled *The Villagers' Friend and Physician* in which he discussed the principles of health and disease, emphasized the importance of exercise and bathing, and stressed the dangers of drinking and overwork. He also recalled the frustrations of unnecessary night calls in stormy weather and suggested consideration for the comfort and wellbeing of the physician of the future!

Amidst all these activities he wrote his *Essay on the Shaking Palsy*, a classic of medical history, accurate observation, and literary style which has justly given him enduring eponymous fame. By careful description and cautious conjecture he was able to separate the illness from other similar disorders of movement, such as the tremor affecting the elderly, and to suggest, in the absence of post-mortem findings, the probable site of the disease.

The occurrence of Parkinson's disease

We now know that Parkinson's disease is a very common ailment. In Northern Europe and the United States at least one in every thousand of the population will develop Parkinson's disease; and for those aged between 60 and 80, the risk is approximately one in a hundred. These figures are approximate and may well underestimate the true frequency: mildly affected individuals may not come to medical attention and other illnesses may simulate the disorder.

The illness appears to be slightly more common in men and about three-quarters of all patients develop the malady between the ages of 50 and 70. Contrary to popular opinion, however, it is not only a disease of old age, and not uncommonly first appears between the ages of 30 and 40.

Parkinson's disease is no respecter of persons, race, or creed, and seems to occur in a similar manner throughout the world. However, its frequency may vary somewhat. For example, it is less common in Nigerians than in blacks living in the deep south of the USA. It seems to be particularly common in children and young adults in Japan. Many people in China and India are affected, but there is a suggestion that it might be a little less common in the Third World. One fascinating fact is that Parkinson's disease occurs twice as often in individuals who have never smoked tobacco. This seems to be unrelated to any protective effects of nicotine, but rather to some pattern of behaviour found in those at risk of getting the illness and also in non-smokers. For example, it has been pointed out that many parkinsonian patients are introverted and slightly obsessional with a tendency to get depressed, whereas cigarette smokers are often extroverted risk-takers. Despite these intriguing speculations, we do not recommend even moderate cigarette smoking as a protection against the malady.

Several neurological diseases masquerade as Parkinson's disease. For most of these so-called Parkinson's syndromes the cause is as cryptic and elusive as for Parkinson's disease itself, but in some cases it is understood. The most common of these Parkinson's syndromes is that caused by the use of a group of powerful drugs used by physicians to treat serious mental illness, dizziness, and dyspepsia. Fortunately, withdrawal of the offending drug usually leads to a gradual disappearance of all symptoms. There are a number of other disorders with ungainly scientific or eponymous names like strio-nigral degeneration, the Steele–Richardson–Olszewski syndrome, corticobasal degeneration, and diffuse cortical Lewy body disease, which may look very like Parkinson's disease but which are distinct diseases needing different treatment. A disorder of copper metabolism called Wilson's disease can present with parkinsonism in the young and can be effectively treated with drugs which remove excess copper from the body. Repeated small strokes can give a picture similar to Parkinson's disease and, exceptionally, water on the brain (hydrocephalus) or a brain tumour may also present in this way.

The nervous system

In order to understand what goes wrong in Parkinson's disease a rudimentary understanding of how the human brain works is required. Essentially, the nervous system consists of complex arrangements of nerve cells and their connections which combine to control and integrate bodily functions so that the whole being can respond in a co-ordinated manner to the outside world. The most sophisticated structure is the cerebrum or the forebrain, composed of two large hemispheres which function as a central sorting exchange. Under the microscope, the cerebral hemispheres can be seen to consist of millions of nerve cells (grey matter) and vast networks of elongated nerve fibres (white matter) which relay information and which are held together by supportive tissue. Behind the cerebrum is the hindbrain or cerebellum and the spinal cord which is connected to the cerebrum by the brain-stem. The brain-stem is an important junction for the processing of nerve messages as it connects with the cerebellum as well as the cerebrum and spinal cord. The latter is about two and a half feet (about three-quarters of a metre) long and is essentially a great trunk of nerve fibres bearing messages. Together these structures make up

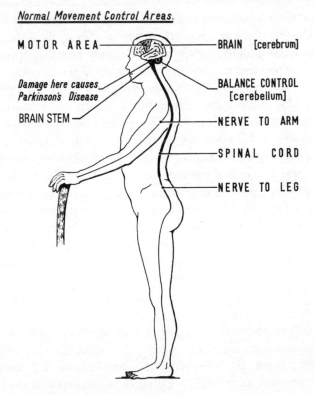

Fig. 1   A simplified plan of the nervous system.

our central nervous system (Fig. 1). The spinal cord nerve cells are in contact with higher centres in the brain and also pass on information through the peripheral nervous system to the rest of our body. This network sends out increasingly fine branches to supply practically every part of the body.

While the whole nervous system is concerned with the control of movement, certain areas have become particularly specialized for this purpose. Many movements are executed without conscious thought. For example, if a child pricks his finger on a drawing-pin his hand is instantaneously withdrawn long before he consciously decides to take protective action. In that brief interval, the pain message has passed from nerve endings in the fingers to the spinal cord and an executive signal of withdrawal has been transmitted to the muscles of the child's hand. These simple but essential actions are carried out by the spinal cord without directly involving the brain. This is called a 'reflex action' and tapping the knee to make the leg jerk is a well-known example. Reflex subconscious responses play a crucial role in modulating and programming patterns of movement. Complex movements, however, require the intervention of higher centres of the nervous system.

In the brain there is a specialized strip of tissue which integrates compound movements organized at lower centres so that skilled and refined motor plans can be carried out. The cerebellum is particularly involved in the control of posture and balance in space and acts as a modulating or braking device on voluntary movement, damping down and preventing excessive overshoot. Finally, there are the basal ganglia, large masses of grey matter located deep in the white substance of the cerebral hemispheres. These are made up of a striped organ (corpus striatum), a smaller pale body (globus pallidus), the triangular thalamus, and a black, pigmented strip of tissue in the brain-stem (substantia nigra). These ganglia and their connections are considered to be part of a primitive motor system which has waned in importance during the course of evolution as the cerebrum has increased in complexity, capacity, and accomplishments. Nevertheless, the basal ganglia are essential programming centres for movement information which is directed from the main motor pathways in the cerebrum. Disturbances in this region of the brain lead to the difficulties patients with

Parkinson's disease have in starting up movements and switching smoothly through a series of separate movements. Although these systems are extraordinarily complex in structure and function, the basic end result of each unit results in excitation or inhibition of the adjacent unit. Many of the dense network of fibres in the central nervous system are inhibitory in function and the normal, smooth, refined actions and complicated tasks depend essentially on interacting feedback loop systems. We all find it difficult to accept that the extraordinary skills of a professional musician can be explained in terms of ganglia, nerve cells, feedback systems, and on–off codes of inhibition and excitation, but, whatever the nature of genius, it requires the same basic neural apparatus to manifest itself.

The site of disturbance of function in Parkinson's disease

When James Parkinson described his disease, examination of affected brains was not possible and he could only hazard a guess at the probable site of disturbance of function. Reasoning from the fact that the disease involved the whole body, he shrewdly speculated that the site of the damage was in the nervous system, more specifically the top of the spinal cord and lower portion of the brain-stem. In the mid-nineteenth century, several patients who had died with Parkinson's disease were examined but no obvious abnormality could be recognized in the nervous system. Indeed, several distinguished authorities wondered whether Parkinson's disease was a functional disorder of the brain akin to depression and anxiety. In 1893, the first breakthrough occurred in Paris. A patient, who during life had Parkinson's disease limited to one side of the body, died and post-mortem examination disclosed a small tumour pressing on the basal ganglia on the opposite side of his brain. The following year, Professor Brissaud suggested that focal damage to the black substance might be the cause. Inspired by this suggestion, a young doctor called Trétiakoff meticulously examined the substantia nigra in nine patients and was rewarded by confirming that the principal symptoms of Parkinson's disease were indeed due to damage to this distinctive strip of black pigment containing nerve cells. These seminal observations are generally accepted although it is now also agreed that other bits of the brain-stem may be damaged too.

If the brain of a patient with Parkinson's disease is examined with the naked eye, the only definite abnormality is loss of black pigment (Plate I). The use of the microscope and sophisticated tissue-staining methods discloses further abnormality. The pigmented nerve cells of the black substance (substantia nigra) are greatly reduced in number and many of the survivors look frail. Some of the degenerating cells contain particles called Lewy bodies consisting of concentric masses of amorphous material with a dark core and a paler halo (Plate II). Demonstration of their presence is as important as finding nerve cell loss in confirming the diagnosis of Parkinson's disease after death. As many as 1 in 10 of 80-year-olds may at the time of death be harbouring these Lewy bodies in their brains, even though there were no signs of Parkinson's disease in life. Many of these individuals also have some loss of nerve cells in the black substance but not enough to lead to the appearance of Parkinson's disease. This suggests that as many as 10 per cent of octagenarians may be 'incubating' Parkinson's disease but because of the very gradual progression of the illness they die from some other cause before it can appear.

The nature of Parkinson's disease

The nerve cell

Attention now has to be directed to the basic unit of nervous tissue, which is called a nerve cell or neuron (Fig. 2). This is too small to be seen by the naked eye, but it is a crucial and complex structure adapted to transmit information rapidly through the brain and around the body. These messages are conducted along the neuron, first by wire-like processes or extensions of the neuron called dendrites, and then down a long, thin tube called an axon. Information is transmitted in the form of electrical charges or impulses which are generated by a series of chemical reactions across the wall or membrane of the neuron. Some axons are insulated with layers of fat-containing material

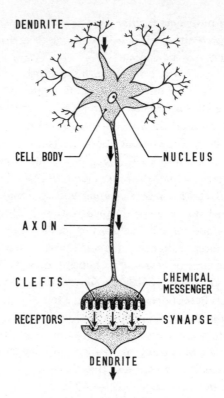

Fig. 2 A typical nerve cell and its connections.

called myelin which permits the electrical charges to travel
more rapidly.

Nerve cells are never in direct physical continuity with one
another but are separated by a small gap called a synapse. When the
electrical impulse reaches the end of an axon it stimulates the
adjacent nerve endings across the synapse by releasing chemical
messengers. These substances are made within the nerve cell and
conveyed to the terminals adjacent to the synapse where they are
stored in small packages. The arrival of the appropriate electrical
trigger at the end of an axon releases some of the chemical
messenger which crosses the gap between the cells (the synapse)
where each molecule latches on tightly to the specific chemical
receptors on the wall of the dendrite of the next cell. Some of the
chemical messenger is destroyed while the rest is retrieved and

stored within the axon for further use. Thus by a combination of electrical and chemical events, information can be rapidly con-veyed from neuron to neuron and hence, throughout the nervous system.

Dopamine—a chemical messenger

The idea that chemical messengers exist in the brain was suspected more than fifty years ago, but confirmation has come only recently since when much has been learned about these neurotransmitters, their function and regulation. So far at least a hundred distinct chemicals which modify nerve function have been isolated and such is the rate of research in this field that new substances are being discovered every year.

By the 1950s, a chemical substance called dopamine was known to be present in the human brain, but it was thought to be a relatively inactive compound whose main function was to produce the 'fight or flight' stress chemicals, adrenalin and noradrenalin. However, when it was found that high concentrations of dopamine were present in parts of the basal ganglia where noradrenalin was virtually absent, it seemed likely that dopamine might have a function of its own. Sensitive and highly selective chemical stains were developed and with these new techniques a group of Swedish scientists were able to demonstrate a pathway between dopamine-containing cells in the substantia nigra and cells in the striped body (corpus striatum) of the basal ganglia. This has become important in our understanding of how Parkinson's disease develops and it is this group of cells and their connecting fibres which the surgeons are attempting to replace in the brain implant experiments.

The connection between dopamine and Parkinson's disease

Progress in science is often dependent upon luck and serendipity and the next phase in unravelling the mysteries of the disease came to pass by a fascinating combination of ancient world medicine and sophisticated scientific technology. The main clues which proved to be crucial in unravelling this mystery, which had many compli-cated twists and turns, were as follows. The extract of a small shrub, *Rauwolfia serpentina*—so called because the classification of this plant with elongated, crooked roots had been attributed to a botanist called Rauwolf—had long been revered in India because of its medicinal properties (Plate III). Reference can be found in ancient Sanskrit incunabula and it is also mentioned in Ayurvedic commentaries as a useful sedative drug. One of its many synonyms is 'chandra' which means 'moon' in Bengali, probably indicating an association with lunacy or madness and the efficacy of this natural medicine. Whatever the origins of the folklore, it was commonly used as a mild, effective sedative and it is recorded that the late Mahatma Gandhi regularly used the plant as an infusion to overcome nervousness and secure a sound night's sleep.

After the Second World War, Indian physicians reported that *Rauwolfia* could reduce high blood pressure and a number of bitter alkaline chemicals called alkaloids were extracted from the roots of the plant and confirmed to have both sedative and blood-pressure-lowering properties. The most active of these substances was named reserpine and within a year of its introduction a most spectacular side-effect was noticed: a condition indistinguishable from Parkinson's disease developed in a few patients. When the drug was discontinued the signs of parkinsonism disappeared. This exciting discovery opened up a new era of research. Arvid Carlsson, a young Swedish scientist, found that when he injected reserpine into rats a state of rigid immobility was produced resembling the severest form of Parkinson's disease. He was able to demonstrate that in the brains of the affected animals there had been a severe depletion of certain chemical substances, including dopamine. He then found that if he gave an injection of levodopa (L-dopa), the chemical precursor of dopamine, to the afflicted rats they recovered rapidly. Clearly dopamine was vitally involved in the regulation of normal movement in the rat. Three years later in Vienna, Oleh Hornykiewicz found the final piece of the jigsaw when he discovered that the brains of people who had died with Parkinson's disease contained very little dopamine.

Supporting evidence for these seminal observations speedily emerged from laboratories all over the world. The relationship of dopamine to Parkinson's disease was intensively studied and it was confirmed beyond all doubt to be a chemical messenger which regulated the release of hormones and influenced mood and behaviour as well as modulating the control of movement (Fig. 3).

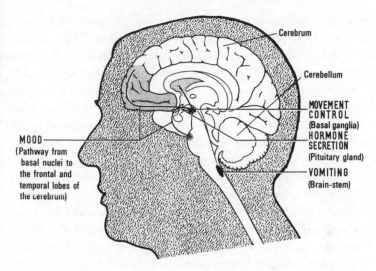

Cerebrum

Cerebellum

MOVEMENT
CONTROL
(Basal ganglia)
HORMONE
SECRETION
(Pituitary gland)

VOMITING
(Brain-stem)

MOOD
(Pathway from
basal nuclei to
the frontal and
temporal lobes of
the cerebrum)

Fig. 3 Body functions influenced by the chemical messenger, dopamine.

The excitement was intense. A degenerative neurological disease of unknown cause could now be explained in terms of chemical changes and the possibility of effective treatment became a reality. As is so often the case, initial impressions were too simple and ingenuous and the story has turned out to be far more complicated, still leaving much to be explained. The fundamental cause of the dopamine deficiency remains a complete mystery and the significance of disturbances in other brain neurotransmitters has still to be elucidated. When this code has been cracked it is very likely that even more effective treatment will become available. Armed with our present knowledge, albeit limited, it is now possible to make some headway in understanding the fundamental mechanisms of the parkinsonian disabilities.

How dopamine deficiency leads to Parkinsonian symptoms

The slowness and poverty of movement (bradykinesia) in Parkinson's disease can be attributed to damage of the bundle of dopamine-containing nerve fibres which connect the substantia nigra and the corpus striatum in the basal ganglia. Damage to these nerve fibres allows unwanted and excessive excitatory messages to escape from the corpus striatum which are transformed in the neighbouring thalamus into oscillating bursts of nervous activity. These are then relayed on through the cerebrum, brainstem, and spinal cord. The oscillating drive of abnormal impulses results in a tremble. Thus, shaking can be considered as an escape or release phenomenon due to impaired efficiency of the normal dampening mechanisms in the nervous system. The muscle stiffness can be explained in terms of an excessive discharge of certain nerve impulses to muscle mechanisms responsible for tone (the normal resistance of the limbs to passive stretch) and, like tremor, it is essentially the consequence of defective inhibitory mechanisms arising in the substantia nigra.

These explanations are probably far too superficial and facile and much remains to be explained. In the years ahead, the mechanisms of movement control in health and disease will receive intensive study in the reasonable expectation that effective treatments will arise from rational explanations. The realization that a hitherto untreatable illness can be explained at least partially in terms of disordered brain chemistry has been a tremendous stimulus to further research and has already brought palpable benefit to thousands of disabled people.

2. What are the symptoms and course of Parkinson's disease?

Symptoms

During the course of the illness—particularly during the early stages when the significance of certain symptoms may not be clear—it may be necessary to resort to certain investigations such as blood tests, X-rays, and brain scans, essentially to exclude other causes. There is no specific laboratory test which becomes positive in the presence of Parkinson's disease: the diagnosis can be made only by consideration of an individual's symptoms and incapacities.

The onset is so gradual that many patients, even with hindsight, may be uncertain when their troubles began. This difficulty may be shared by close relatives and friends who may fail to notice slow changes in appearance; paradoxically those who see the patient infrequently may be immediately struck by altered facial expression, quality of voice, posture, or physical alacrity. It is a strange irony that the patient may be completely unaware of changes in himself which would be immediately evident to a stranger. Early symptoms may be vague and non-specific: inexplicable tiredness and lassitude, unwarranted fatiguability, mild muscular aches and cramps, vague tingling or pins and needles, can easily be misconstrued by patients and also by experienced doctors as evidence of strain, overwork, or mild depression. To compound this difficulty, puzzled and frustrated by insidious and inexplicable malaise, the patient may become genuinely depressed by increasing incapacity. This difficulty—of distinguishing between physical and psychological symptoms—can be further complicated by the patient's expressionless and unresponsive appearance. The 'mask-like' face (often a feature of Parkinson's disease) not only dampens down the normal indications of feeling such as a wry smile or grimace which are part of the normal physical language of communication, but may erroneously indicate loss of interest, withdrawal, or rejection, provoking consequent distress to relatives and friends. Gradually, more specific difficulties emerge. These are often first noticed in the hands. Writing may become progressively smaller, irregular, less legible, and more laborious. Sentences tend to drift across the page and may merge into an indecipherable scrawl. One patient shrewdly demonstrated the insidious onset of his illness over many years and subsequently his beneficial response to treatment by flicking through the stubs of previous cheque books. The initial clarity, deterioration, then subsequent improvement on treatment, vividly illustrated the stages of his illness.

Increasing slowness and impaired dexterity for skilled tasks (particularly for those involving rapid, repetitive movements) gradually become evident in a host of minor personal habits. For example, a conscious effort may become necessary to cope with previously automatic chores such as stirring a cup of tea, cleaning the teeth, shaving, and coping with buttons, cufflinks, or jewellery. Women often recall that one of the earliest difficulties is fixing the clip of a bra between the shoulders; men frequently mention the exasperation of coping with their top shirt button. One man repeatedly returned a self-winding watch to the manufacturer before he appreciated that his own sluggish wrist movements were responsible. Early difficulties may be so idiosyncratic that those whose occupations involve skilled manual tasks may be long aware of subtle physical impediment before a doctor can confirm this in the course of his physical examination. However, remarkable individual exceptions occur. Thus, a morse-code operator confidently maintained his exacting signalling speeds while his handwriting showed unequivocal deterioration; a housewife could still play the piano well whilst being obliged to give up embroidery; a professional clavicord player had difficulty in dressing yet could perform competently in public.

A special effort may become necessary to rise from a familiar chair and, with hindsight, may be the first unequivocal milestone of increasing incapacity. A customary stroll usually accomplished in a relaxed, effortless manner may be disturbed by heaviness or slight dragging of one leg which may not be evident to a skilled observer over short distances. Thus, early in the course of the illness when these subtle changes are occurring there may be little or nothing for the doctor to discover despite a meticulous physical examination. Further time may have to elapse before evidence of one or more of the classic signs—tremor, rigidity, or bradykinesia (explained below)—becomes evident and the diagnosis can be firmly established.

The classical symptoms of Parkinson's disease

Tremor—a pattern of shaking defined as an involuntary rhythmical movement of small amplitude

This is the most conspicuous sign and although embarrassing paradoxically it often proves to be the least disabling. At some stage it affects the majority of patients and because it is such an obvious departure from normal it is usually the symptom which brings the patient to his family doctor. Many patients describe an awareness of internal tremulousness long before the appearance of overt shaking that is recognizable by others. Tremor usually begins in one hand, less often in a foot, and only rarely in the lips or jaw. As James Parkinson shrewdly noted there is a characteristic tendency for tremor to occur when the affected limb is at rest and to diminish or disappear during voluntary movements. This is not invariably so: some patients have tremor during active movements such as bringing a teacup to their lips. The frequency of the tremor is about five times a second and this helps to distinguish it from other causes such as anxiety or over-activity of the thyroid gland which causes a much finer, faster movement. While tremor may be limited to one finger, more often it involves all the fingers and the thumb, sometimes provoking a to-and-fro oscillation of the thumb against the index finger which early physicians, accustomed to preparing their medications by hand, called 'pill rolling'. In the early stages, tremor may be present only for short periods when the individual is weary or fatigued or during times of emotional stress. Even at later stages, the tremble may fluctuate very considerably in intensity, duration, and extent, so that at times the whole of the limb is vigorously involved and yet within the space of seconds no tremor can be seen. On occasions severe, incapacitating tremor which has troubled a patient for months and sometimes years, may completely resolve. These variations may be totally unpredictable, but exacerbation by stress and relief during relaxation is the rule. Tremor markedly diminishes during deep sleep, but observant spouses report that movements can be seen from time to time perhaps related to vivid dreams or lightness of sleep.

Many patients firmly date the onset of tremor to a particularly distressing personal event such as bereavement, a business setback, or an accident. While it is extremely unlikely that there is a direct cause-and-effect interpretation, the importance of emotional factors in enhancing latent tremor cannot be denied. Many become adept in disguising tremor of one hand by assuming a Napoleonic posture or literally sitting on the problem during an interview; a few are able, at least for short periods, to inhibit shaking by an intense effort of will power. All are deeply concerned about the consequences of an easily recognizable disability which can be misunderstood by others, particularly when their livelihood might be affected. They know all too well that the brusque reactions of an unsympathetic employer, dissatisfied customer, or an irascible colleague can make a mild tremor considerably worse, which in turn provokes agitation and a vicious cycle of tremor and worry. Rest tremor which disappears during action rarely affects the performance of skilled tasks. In the early days of stereotactic surgery (this will be discussed further in Chapter 4), it was often possible to suppress tremor dramatically after a successful operation, and yet patients ruefully remarked that they could do little more with their hands than they could before surgery. This is because the other components of parkinsonism were still present.

Rigidity—a stiffness of muscles and joints recognized by the examiner by increased resistance to passive movements of a limb, such as the wrist, elbow, or knee

Because it was not, at that time, customary to examine patients in detail, James Parkinson made no mention of rigidity which causes muscles to move more slowly and which may give rise to cramps, aches, and stiffness. These may be so distressing that fibrositis and muscular rheumatism may initially be diagnosed. When the individual's joints are passively moved and the affected muscles stretched, smooth, increased resistance can be detected—likened to bending a lead pipe—but curiously this is rarely noticed by the patient. To the examiner, however, there can be little doubt about the increased resistance to passive movements and frequently there may also be a regular rhythmical jerking quality which has been called 'cogwheel rigidity'. Rigidity can predominantly affect the arm and leg on one side of the body, or it may symmetrically involve all four limbs. The extent and severity of rigidity varies considerably from one individual to another but can almost always be provoked or made more conspicuous when other limbs are vigorously moved. This stratagem is sometimes employed by the doctor when he wants to bring out rigidity when its presence is in doubt. The wrist, for example, is passively flexed and extended while the opposite arm is waved vigorously: a striking increase in rigidity or cogwheeling is usually evident to both patient and examiner.

Bradykinesia

This is a comprehensive term used to describe slowness and poverty of willed movements and also includes delay in initiation as well as difficulty in performing rapid, repetitive tasks and fatiguability. It is the most incapacitating of all the disabilities encountered in Parkinson's disease. It may occur in the absence of rigidity and provide the basis for many of the frustrating difficulties encountered by patients. Reference has already been made to problems such as slowness in dressing, shaving, or stirring tea, but bradykinesia also underlies facial immobility, infrequent blinking, paucity of normal gesture, and grace of expression. Particularly striking, to relatives if not the sufferer, is the impairment or loss of certain spontaneous automatic movements such as the failure to swing the arms symmetrically when walking. This enforced limitation of movement at the shoulder causes secondary stiffening of the joint capsule with localized pain called pericapsulitis or 'frozen shoulder'. Characteristic gestures, mannerisms, and postures which are so idiosyncratic and personal and essential to speech and communication become sluggish, and the normal flow of restlessness and slight fidgetiness—which few of us normally notice when present—such as adjusting clothes, clearing the throat, moving the eyes and the head, may be conspicuous by their absence. Fortunately, bradykinesia responds well to medical treatment.

With the passage of time, and it must be emphasized that these comments apply mainly to the unrecognized and untreated disorder, it is often difficult to be sure whether a patient's incapacities are primarily due to increasing rigidity, bradykinesia, or separate obstacles to normal movement such as disordered balance and posture. For example, there is a gradual postural tendency towards a position of flexion: the chin tends to bend towards the chest; the shoulders become rounded; the arms flexed at the elbows; and the knees tend to be held in a slightly bent position not only when upright but also when reclining in bed. When walking, the patient is inclined to lean forwards, the general pattern of gait becomes less springy, the length of pace shortens, and steps may become increasingly rapid, so that a characteristic shuffle emerges (Fig. 4). Turning in confined spaces may require a series of fragmented hesitant manoeuvres. Occasionally, both feet seem to be stuck to the ground and there may be a distressing delay before walking can be initiated. This 'freezing' may occur in a capricious and unpredictable manner, but there is a particular tendency for it to happen when moving from one room to another or when attempting to suddenly change direction. Some patients are able to walk effortlessly on grass, pebbles, and uneven surfaces, but tend to seize up on paving stones, or stairs, or other smooth areas; other patients report the converse.

The muscles which determine the quality and clarity of the voice may become involved so that speech becomes slower, muffled, and quiet. The normal fall and rise of the voice in animated conversation becomes dampened and the rhythm of speech assumes a monotonous quality. Paradoxically, in certain individuals speech becomes faster and, as a consequence, difficult to comprehend. The same group of muscles are involved in the automatic mechanisms of swallowing mucus and saliva. When healthy, we rarely think about this drainage mechanism except perhaps when sitting in the dentist's chair and we are prevented from moving the lower jaw and coping with the normal accretion of saliva. In Parkinson's disease the volume of saliva is not increased, but when the

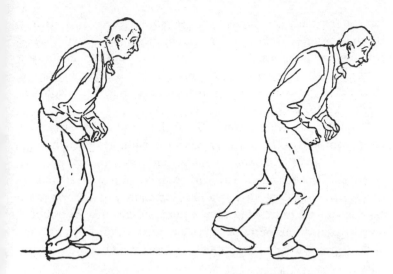

Fig. 4   A drawing by Paul Richer to show the posture and 'hurrying' gait of advanced Parkinson's disease.

mechanisms are slowed down by ridigity or immobility, dribbling occurs.

Intellectual changes

James Parkinson wrote that 'throughout the course of the illness the senses and intellect were preserved'. While this remains true for most patients, we now know that when parkinsonism has been present for many years about 30 per cent show changes in intellect and personality. Such changes are usually slight and only evident to those who know the individual well. Memory for day-to-day events may become less reliable and there may be greater difficulty in putting names to faces than we usually accept with advancing years. More noticeable may be a loss of drive, enthusiasm, and curiosity. More time may be spent passively watching television than reading books and newspapers and perhaps, partly as a consequence, the content of conversation becomes less stimulating and lively. Rarely, intellectual changes become more conspicuous: fading concentration and inattentiveness may pass gradually to disorientation and intermittent confusion. Some of these changes can be partially attributed to the side-effects of medicines employed, some to the fact that patients with Parkinson's disease are now living a normal life-span and natural ageing changes are taking toll, but in a few patients brain changes beyond the basal ganglia and movement control mechanisms must be accepted as part of the disease process.

While these observations about the gradual evolution of parkinsonian disabilities over the course of time are generally true, there is a great individual variation in pattern, cadence, and severity. Certain individuals with a predominantly tremulous illness may show little deterioration over many years, others never experience a tremble, while some young patients may be troubled only by contortions of the feet for many years before other features of the illness emerge. Each patient is a law unto himself.

3. What is the cause of Parkinson's disease?

One hundred years ago Brissaud, a French neurologist, wrote that 'Parkinson's disease remains so utterly inexplicable that we are constantly drawn to it by the lure of the mysterious'. Unfortunately, his sentiment can be echoed today. Despite intensive research there remains a dearth of solid facts on which to base even reasonable speculations, and the fashionable notions of today will undoubtedly prove to be as ludicrous and naïve as those so vehemently espoused by our predecessors. For instance, Parkinson himself considered rheumatism and bowel inflammation to be important, whereas Victorian puritanism led to the firm conviction that sexual over-indulgence was at the root of the malady. Charcot was impressed by the frequency with which the disorder followed stressful events or physical injury, whereas, up to quite recently, deficient blood supply to the brain was believed to be the commonest cause in the elderly.

One of the most durable theories has been that put forward by one of the founders of British neurology, Gowers, who first suggested that areas of the nervous system wear out at different rates so that one man will prematurely lose his balance, another his intellectual power, and a third the black substance of the midbrain causing Parkinson's disease. This is an attractive if somewhat simple hypothesis because some of the features of the illness are reminiscent of the disorders of movement seen in extreme old age. For instance, an actor simulating an elderly person will often stoop, shuffle, tremble, and assume a reedy, hesitant speech. Even if this abiotrophy theory should be proved to be correct, it provides only a partial and insubstantial answer to the enigma, and spawns a new cluster of imponderable questions. For example, how important are hereditary factors or previous cryptic environmental insults in predisposing certain individuals to the disease? Does the body produce toxins which damage its own nerve cells and if so how are they scavenged normally? These are some of the difficult conundrums occupying scientists throughout the world who, every day, try to bring us nearer to understanding. Even the discovery of further intermediate biological abnormalities could lead to efficacious preventative therapies. For example, if a toxin, MPTP, which has been found to cause parkinsonism in Californian drug addicts is relevant to the aetiology of Parkinson's disease, then selegiline (deprenyl), a drug used to treat the disorder and which prevents MPTP toxicity in animals, might also curtail the disease process if given early enough. At the present time, however, this remains no more than idle conjecture.

The rest of this chapter outlines contemporary dogma. One can only hope that a judicious fusion of good fortune, methodical clinical research, and painstaking basic science will soon throw up vital new leads which will take us a few steps further forward. Physicians must remain open to all new suggestions and patients and their carers must communicate their ideas on the cause however fanciful they may seem.

Is it an inherited condition?

Many people with Parkinson's disease know of an aunt or uncle with similar symptoms, but the relationship is usually distant. Only rarely is a parent, brother, or sister affected. There are a few exceptional families in which several generations have been affected. These must be clearly distinguished from the common familial disease known as essential tremor whose members have a tremor but do not have Parkinson's disease (whether an association exists between essential tremor and Parkinson's disease is still not clear). If inheritance is an important factor, identical twins, who receive the same genetic material from their parents, should both show a similar tendency to inherit parkinsonism. In fact this does not seem to happen. In one study of 37 pairs of twins of whom one had Parkinson's disease, in only two cases was the other twin affected. The highly sophisticated method of tissue typing, currently used to match organs for transplantation, has failed to reveal

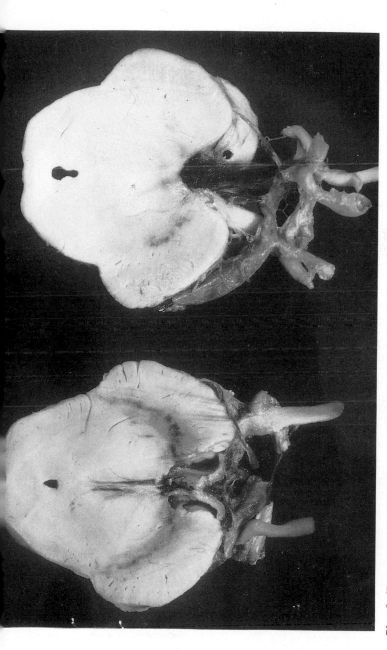

Plate I. Transverse sections of the upper part of the human hind brain showing the loss of black pigment in a patient with Parkinson's disease contrasted with a normal pigmented control.

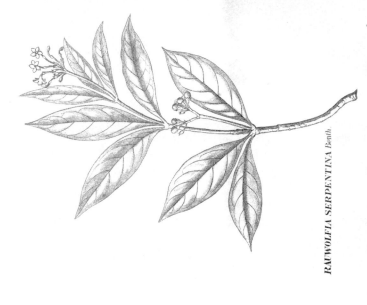

RAUWOLFIA SERPENTINA Benth.

Plate III. *Rauwolfia serpentina*, a natural source of reserpine which can cause drug-induced Parkinsonism.

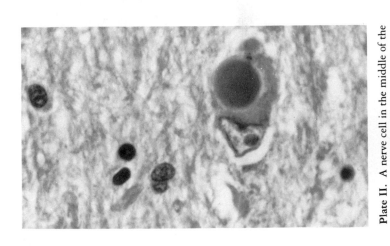

Plate II. A nerve cell in the middle of the picture showing a large circular Lewy body with a paler halo around it (X 800).

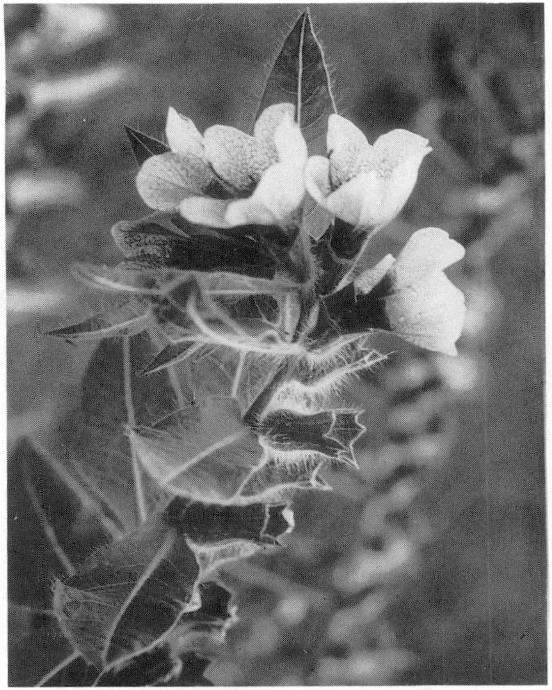

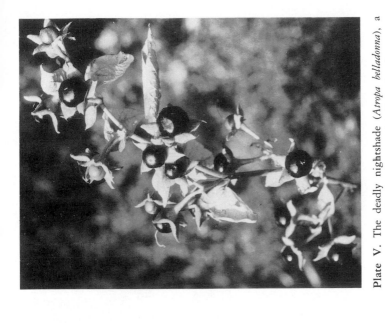

Plate IV. The black henbane (*Hyoscyamus niger*), a rich source of the anticholinergic medicine hyoscyamine.

Plate V. The deadly nightshade (*Atropa belladonna*), a natural source of atropine, an anticholinergic substance.

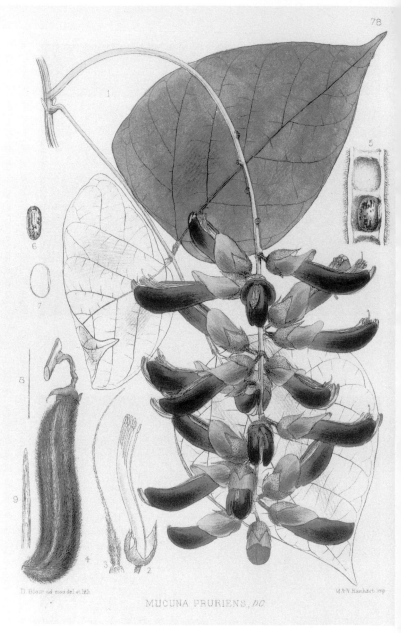

Plate VI. The cowhage, *Mucuna pruriens*, a natural source of L-dopa.

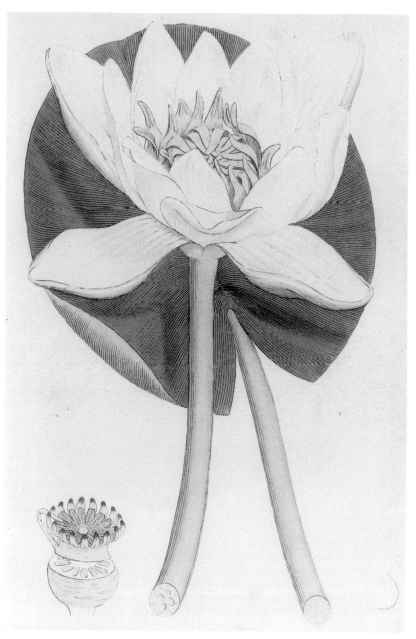

Plate VII. The waterlily, *Nymphaea alba*, a natural source of apomorphine.

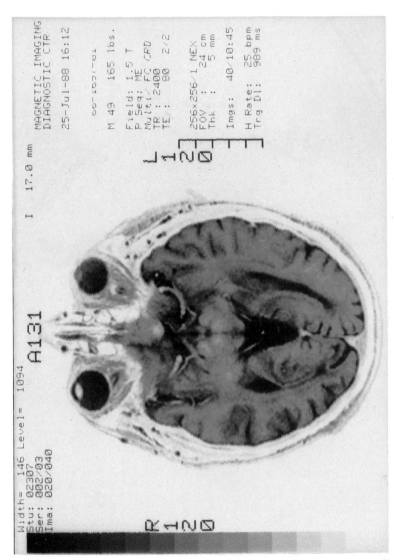

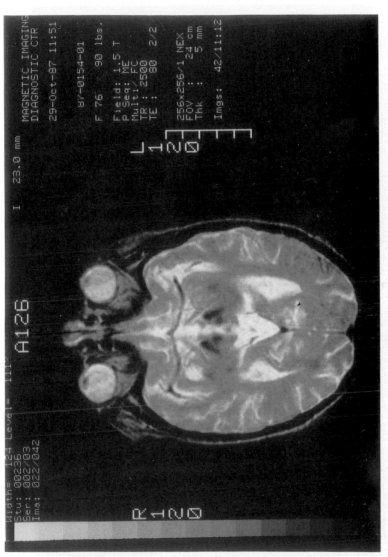

Plate VIII. MRI scan showing (a) normal anatomy of substantia nigra and (b) decreased size of substantia nigra in Parkinson's disease.

(b)

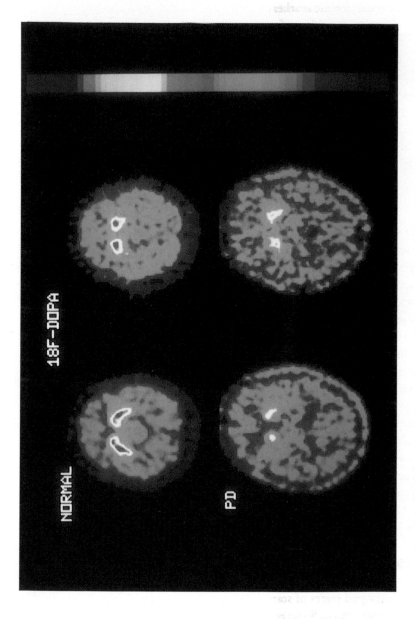

Plate IX. A PET scan depicting a deficiency of L-dopa in the brain of a Parkinsonian compared to a control.

any particular genetic marker or vulnerability to the disease. Thus, while the present evidence for recognizable inheritance for parkinsonism remains inconclusive, it can be firmly stated that the risk of transmitting the illness to one's children is extremely small. Parkinson's disease is not an hereditary disorder such as haemophilia or Huntington's chorea, where the risks are considerable and can be calculated with accuracy. It is just conceivable that there is something in the basic physical make-up of people with Parkinson's disease which renders them susceptible to the illness, but it is not an inherited condition in the normal sense of the word.

Is it due to a virus?

In the winter of 1916–17, a strange new illness appeared in Vienna and spread throughout the world during the next decade. The symptoms were wide-ranging. Many patients fell into a prolonged, unrouseable stupor, with paralysis of eye movements; others became delirious and experienced insomnia so severe that sedation was ineffectual. Successive winters brought thousands of new victims. Constantin von Economo, a Viennese physician, established that despite their variable symptomatology all the patients had the same disease, which became known as the sleeping sickness or epidemic encephalitis lethargica. Von Economo was able to show that all the patients who died had the same pattern of damage to the brain and that the illness could be transmitted to monkeys by inoculation. This strongly suggested an infective agent was responsible even though it could not be identified under the microscope. The epidemic raged on, killing many and leaving thousands of brain-damaged survivors, until 1927–28 when the illness disappeared as mysteriously as it had come. Few patients recovered completely. Some were so apathetic, inert, and withdrawn that they were likened to 'spent volcanoes', suspended in time, unable to remain in contact with the outside world. Children were transformed into rebellious anti-social delinquents. Many adults developed states of statuesque rigidity comparable to those seen in schizophrenia. Some echoed whatever was said to them, developed obsessional and bizarre mannerisms, hallucinations, and even dancing movements. In addition to this extraordinary catalogue, many patients developed an unusual form of Parkinson's disease. This could develop within a few weeks of the infection, but could be delayed for as long as 30 years. The illness was atypical in many respects including an unusual phenomenon when the eyes would be forcibly and uncontrollably deviated upwards or to one side, often for several hours, so-called oculogyric crisis. This could also be accompanied by intense flushing of the face, confusion, and emotional excitement. Fortunately, there has been no recurrence of this dreadful epidemic and most of the survivors with post-encephalitic parkinsonism are now in their seventies. Many were confined to long-stay institutions as children and have remained there ever since. A vivid and moving account of a community of post-encephalitic patients in Mount Carmel Hospital, New York, was drawn by Dr Oliver Sacks in his remarkable book *Awakenings*. A similar colony exists in the UK at Highlands Hospital in North London. The resilience and enduring cheerfulness of these survivors is an extraordinary tribute to the human spirit.

While the features of the epidemic strongly suggest that a transmissible agent was culpable, intensive research at that time, and subsequently, failed to incriminate a particular bacteria, virus, or infectious agent as the cause of the Parkinson's disease arising from this illness. Epidemiological evidence culled from a study of causes of death as recorded on contemporary death certificates indicates that people born between 1880 and 1900 had a higher mortality from Parkinson's disease throughout the period 1931–75 than people born before or after that time. This is consistent with the hypothesis that people likely to have been exposed to encephalitis lethargica (that is those aged between 20 and 40 in 1920) had a higher rate of mortality from Parkinson's disease than others. This could be interpreted as support to the possibility of a viral infective cause for some cases of Parkinson's disease today. The mystery persists despite the development of modern techniques to isolate and cultivate viruses from human tissue.

Despite theoretical speculation there is no evidence that poliomyelitis or rheumatic fever can lead to the illness. Very rarely, we still see a patient who develops an encephalitic illness which is followed by the development of atypical parkinsonism. The presumptive evidence that the brain infection was due to a virus is very persuasive, but it is exceptional to identify the responsible agent accurately. Perhaps we have not been looking for the right organism or perhaps there are transmissible factors that we do not yet recognize, but clearly it is important that the search must continue using the tools of modern microbiological research.

Can it be caused by environmental poisons, dietary deficiencies, or drugs?

There are a few chemicals used in industry, and occasionally in the home, which can, very rarely, cause Parkinson's syndrome. Poisoning with coal gas (carbon monoxide), carbon disulphide (an organic solvent used in the rubber industry), potassium cyanide, and methyl alcohol have all been reported. Manganese miners of Chile, India, and Africa who are exposed to long-term inhalation of ore dust may develop an illness resembling parkinsonism with painful spasms and unusual emotional reactions. Mercury poisoning (the hatters' shakes) causes a fine tremor, but this is different in character from that which occurs in Parkinson's disease. It must be stressed, however, that these recognizable causes account for only a tiny minority of parkinsonian illnesses and despite intensive research no noxious substances have been found which could explain the development of the illness in most patients. Extremely sensitive techniques capable of detecting subtle increases in concentrations of trace elements in soil and water have been employed, but as yet no definite environmental link can be demonstrated. Obviously, exposure to modern industrial hazards such as petrol fumes, insecticides, and nuclear waste cannot provide the whole answer as the disease was recognized long before these appeared.

With respect to dietary hazards, the illness occurs in populations eating widely different diets and no particular foodstuff has been incriminated. People who eat roughly the same diet for many years, such as husband and wife or patients confined to long-stay institutions, do not show any increased vulnerability to the illness. It has recently been suggested that prisoners of war who were interned in the Far East and suffered great physical and nutritional neglect may, in later life, show an increased vulnerability to certain chronic neurological diseases including parkinsonism, but the significance remains controversial. For example, some of these individuals may have fallen ill with an encephalitic illness; certainly intercurrent infections in states of profound malnutrition are very common.

In the Mariana islands of the South Pacific (particularly the island of Guam), on the Kii peninsula of Japan, and in Western New Guinea, a special type of Parkinson's syndrome is found which is associated, often in the same individual, with Alzheimer's dementia and motor neuron disease (or amyotrophic lateral sclerosis). Twenty years ago, as many as 1 in 10 of the Chamorro Indians of Guam died from this disease, but it is now less common and whereas formerly it was more common in men it now affects both sexes equally. The cause for this Parkinson–dementia illness is not known, but two theories are of current interest. First, a chronic deficiency of calcium in the diet may lead to an increased absorption of toxic metals like aluminium from the intestine resulting in their abnormal deposition in the brain. Alternatively consumption of a poisonous seed *Cycad circinalis* (false sago palm) used to make bread may be responsible. Although this disease is quite different from Parkinson's disease, if the cause can be unravelled it may help us to understand why nerve cells can be selectively damaged.

It is now clearly recognized that certain drugs and medicines are an increasingly common cause of a pattern of Parkinson's disease indistinguishable from the illness which occurs in the absence of such medications. Powerful tranquillizers, which are extremely effective and valuable in containing serious mental disease, are the chief offenders. There are now many drugs within this group, but the most commonly prescribed are chlorpromazine (Largactil), haloperidol (Serenace, Haldol), thioridazine (Melleril), pimozide (Orap), trifluoperazine (Stelazine), flupenthixol (Depixol), fluphenazine (Modecate), prochlorperazine (Stemetil, Compazine), and flunarizine. All these medications act by fastening on to certain specific chemical receptors in the brain, thereby blocking normal chemical transmission in dopamine pathways which are essential for the control of movement. Fortunately, in most cases, the withdrawal of the tranquillizer leads to slow but complete recovery

from this pattern of parkinsonism. Occasionally, complete resolu-
tion does not occur and it is then presumed that the medicine
unmasks latent Parkinson's disease. The same group of drugs can
also produce other kinds of movement disorders including extreme
physical restlessness, painful spasms of the jaw, tongue and eyes,
and, after sustained treatment, a bizarre condition in which
grimacing, lip-smacking, and tongue protrusion cause great
embarrassment. This latter group of unwanted movements is col-
lectively known as tardive dyskinesia and closely resembles the jerky
movements which occur when exessive amounts of levodopa
are taken. Unlike levodopa-induced movements, tardive dyskinesia
does not always abate when the tranquillizer is reduced or stopped.

Minor, but equally useful, tranquillizing drugs such as diazepam (Valium), chlordiazepoxide (Librium), and the commonly
prescribed medications for insomnia do not cause Parkinson's
disease. Antidepressant drugs are equally blameless.

A more disturbing drug-cause of Parkinson's disease was reported about 6 years ago in a group of narcotic addicts living in the
Bay area of San Francisco. These unfortunate individuals had all
bought a street designer narcotic, MPPP, from a kitchen-chemist.
The batch had been sloppily prepared and contained another
substance, MPTP. This chemical is strikingly similar in composi-
tion to the herbicide Paraquat and was in fact briefly marketed as a
weed-killer. MPTP is converted in the brain to a compound called
MPP^+ which selectively destroys groups of nerve cells and causes
acute, severe, irreversible Parkinson's syndrome in man and be-
havioural disturbances similar to parkinsonism in monkeys.
Although there are minor differences between this drug-induced
disorder and the spontaneously occurring illness, the striking
similarities have excited researchers and led to the suggestion that
there may be environmental toxins, akin to MPTP, which could
cause Parkinson's disease.

Is it due to stressful life events?

All patients and relatives recognize that anxiety and stress tempor-
arily worsen the symptoms of the illness. This is quite different
from suggesting that emotional factors are the primary cause.

Many people definitely date the onset of their illness to a specific emotional upset such as a bereavement. Others refer to a preceding period of wretched depression. At one time it was thought that patients with Parkinson's disease had obsessional personalities and took a rigid, moralistic attitude to life. These sweeping generalizations have no scientific substance whatsoever, although slight mental inflexibility may be a feature of the illness itself. However, doctors have been impressed by the frequency of longstanding depression in many patients with Parkinson's disease; indeed the superficial similarity of the conditions—emotional and physical retardation—has given rise to much thoughtful speculation. The resemblance may be more than superficial because an alkaloid extracted from a plant called *Rauwolfia serpentina* can cause depression in some people, Parkinson's disease in others, and has the biochemical effect of reducing the concentration of a substance called dopamine in the brain (see p. 9). It is therefore conceivable that chronic depression might be associated with depletion of dopamine in the brain which, in turn, might cause parkinsonism. A previous history of depression could be construed as an early warning that brain dopamine levels are diminishing. The hinterland between psychiatric and neurological diseases is currently under intense scrutiny by research workers throughout the world, and from this course advances in our knowledge of chemical reactions within the brain might provide a crucial clue to the cause of parkinsonism.

Could it be due to physical injury?

Repeated serious head injuries can cause numerous small haemorrhages throughout the brain, including the basal ganglia, which, in turn, can cause tremor, rigidity, and physical slowness. This is well-recognized in punch-drunk boxers who, over the course of many years, have prided themselves on their ability to absorb frequent intense physical punishment with consequent irreversible brain damage. They become slow, tremulous, and unsteady, speech is slurred and there are usually profound personality changes. This condition is quite distinct from Parkinson's disease and there is no convincing evidence to suggest that a single head injury, no matter how severe, can account for the subsequent and late development of parkinsonism. Furthermore, most patients with the illness have no antecedent history of significant head injury. Patients commonly date the onset of their illness to a surgical operation, but, assuming that there were no major surgical or anaesthetic catastrophes at the time, it is much more likely that an operation is a significant milestone in anyone's life and there is an understandable tendency to relate the onset of an insidious and otherwise inexplicable incapacity to a definite physical event. Intriguing anecdotes abound of physical injury to one part of the body followed within a short spell of time by signs of Parkinson's disease restricted to the site of injury. It seems probable, if these tantalizing observations are relevant at all, that the local trauma may unmask rather than cause the malady.

The question of accumulation of subtle biochemical injury is extremely difficult to evaluate. For example, there are certain illnesses such as pernicious anaemia and under-activity of the thyroid gland where it is believed that the body produces substances which damage its own tissues (auto-antibodies). The organ singled out for this assault is treated as though it was a foreign tissue and antibodies are produced which attempt to reject and destroy it. This disease process is called 'auto-immune' and, using special techniques, auto-antibodies can be detected in the blood. As yet, none have been found that might damage the dopamine cells of the brain, but, as this is an expanding field of research and much more has to be learned, the possibilities of an auto-immune disturbance as a cause for Parkinson's disease cannot be firmly ruled out. Along similar lines, another intriguing but unproven notion is that in parkinsonism the brain generates a chemical substance related to dopamine which is capable of destroying nerve cells. Substances with these suicidal properties are already known and are utilized in animal research, but they have not yet been found in the brains of patients with Parkinson's disease.

Summary

The age of computers and sophisticated investigative techniques has witnessed great advances in the medical sciences. Cardiac pacemakers, test-tube babies, and organ transplantation, which a generation ago sounded like fantasies of science fiction have become everyday reality. To a considerable extent, research into Parkinson's disease has benefited from similar technological developments, but because of its intrinsic complexity the central nervous system is the most difficult citadel to storm. Scraps of potentially important scientific information relating to mechanisms of brain damage and function continue to accummulate. At present, our understanding of Parkinson's disease remains rudimentary and we are obliged to consider and evaluate any speculation no matter how improbable until the fundamental mechanisms are understood. At present, therefore we know that there are three causes of parkinsonism: (i) a drug-induced reversible disease as a consequence of taking certain medicines, (ii) onset following an inflammatory disease of the brain, or (iii) onset after intoxication with certain industrial poisons. However, these account for only a small minority of patients with parkinsonian disease: for the vast majority of sufferers the primary cause is as cryptic today as it was in James Parkinson's time.

4. What is the treatment?

In the century following the publication of James Parkinson's essay many empirical treatments were recommended for spurious reasons. The discovery of effective measures was initially extremely slow and laborious, but has, fortunately, accelerated with frenetic speed in the past three decades. It is salutary to consider some of the discarded treatments so that the achievements of the modern era can be fully appreciated. James Parkinson warned his readers against precipitous use of irrational therapy, but in the manner of his time resorted to the application of vesicatories to the neck and vigorous blood letting. Other physicians recommended salts of iron, potassium, and barium, and popular palliative measures included narcotic concoctions of cannabis, opium, and arsenic. Calabar beans, purgatives, the rye fungus, hemlock, parathyroid gland extracts, and strychnine had many influential adherents. Others favoured complex elixirs of life, containing substances such as lecithin, phytin, and phosphorus—which are still added to proprietary health foods—and in addition there were secret sera and mysterious animal glandular extracts. This was the era when panaceas and nostrums were fraudulently dispensed to the gullible public by itinerant charlatans and salesmen. Totally unjustified claims of efficacy unfortunately continue. For example, reports of the benefit of insulin injections, hormones, antibiotics, and folic acid have required careful scientific assessment, so dramatic was the alleged benefit. Several times a year a new 'cure' is still publicized by the media. Whether it be supplements of zinc, tin, iron, or the adherence to strange diets or food fads, such unfounded claims provoke great interest and anxiety. It has been justly said that any medicine will improve Parkinson's disease, providing the drug is enthusiastically prescribed and taken. Alas such a response—the so-called placebo effect—is brief. To convincingly demonstrate that a new medicine is truly effective requires carefully planned trials patiently observed for many months.

In the absence of effective medicines physical treatments were often tried. In Paris, Professor Charcot, the most distinguished clinician of his time, was so impressed by the improvement following rides in bumpy, horsedrawn carriages that he constructed a 'fauteuil trépidant' (vibrating chair) in his consulting rooms. Patients sat and shook for fixed periods of time. Osbert Sitwell is reputed to have said that the vibration on a train was as good as two cocktails for improving his parkinsonian tremor. Some of our patients have also reported temporary benefit after bus rides and one man of great technical ingenuity devised a portable vibratory apparatus and gains relief by massaging himself several times a day. Scientists have studied the effects of vibration on movement and have demonstrated that resistance to stretching in muscles may be reduced by certain high frequency stimuli. Perhaps some of the discarded treatments and clinical anecdotes may not be so outrageous after all.

Unfortunately, the era of speculative therapeutics offered little worthwhile benefit for the majority of patients and Parkinson's disease continued to have a grave outlook. Alfred Lord Tennyson was only too well aware of the prospects when he wrote in his poem 'The Two Voices' 'What drug can make a withered palsy cease to shake?'. By the turn of the century the limitations of unconventional measures were appreciated and physicians were offering more realistic advice. Eminent German neurologists, such as Erb and Oppenheim, advised their patients to abstain from cranky diets and to eat simple, nourishing, and varied food. They stressed the importance of reducing undue excitement and emotional stress and encouraged massage, moderate outdoor exercise in the summer, and suggested systems of indoor gymnastics. These sound principles remain applicable today.

Anticholinergic medication

The first intimation of useful medical treatment came in 1880 from Professor Charcot and his colleagues working in the Salpêtrière, a large city asylum for incurables. Ancient folklore described how certain plants could cause the mouth to become dry and Charcot and his colleagues shrewdly exploited this, initially to alleviate the drooling of saliva. Serendipitously they discovered that improvement might also occur in stiffness and trembling. Initially, alcohol extracts from herbs and plants such as black henbane (*Hyoscyamus niger*) (Plate IV) and thorn apple (*Datura stramonium*) were prescribed. The deadly nightshade (*Atropa belladonna*) (Plate V) which had been used for centuries as a natural cosmetic to dilate the pupil of the eye—presumably to render it more alluring—was later found to have similar benefits. The relative merits of these differing preparations culminated in international dispute. 'The Bulgarian belladonna treatment', introduced by a plant collector Ivan Raeff, gained an unwarranted reputation although it contained no more than an elixir of belladonna supplemented by white wine, charcoal, bread dough, sawdust, and nutmeg; but there was substance in these claims and it is fascinating to reflect that the efficacy, albeit limited, of this group of drugs was established long before the scientific basis of their actions was elucidated. Elaborate remedies were gradually replaced by the essential pure alkaloids atropine, hyoscine, and hyoscyamine, and these were taken dissolved in alcohol as tinctures or smoked in cigarette form with tobacco.

About 40 years ago similar synthetically prepared medications with fewer side-effects were introduced and these remain in general use. Those most frequently prescribed in the UK are benzhexol (Artane) and orphenadrine (Disipal); benztropine (Cogentin), procyclidine (Kemadrin), methixene (Tremonil), benapryzine (Brizin), and biperiden (Akineton) are similar drugs. Initial claims of spectacular improvement were wildly exaggerated, but we now know that these agents do offer a modest reduction in rigidity, tremor, and occasionally ameliorate painful cramps. It used to be popular to give combinations of these anticholinergic drugs in small doses, but there is no evidence that this produces greater benefit than one medicine in an appropriate dose. All the anticholinergic drugs work by blocking the reaction of a chemical messenger of neurotransmission called acetylcholine. This has an opposing action to dopamine and so in Parkinson's disease, where there is a deficiency of dopamine, a relative predominance of acetylcholine exists. Anticholinergic drugs are given to redress the

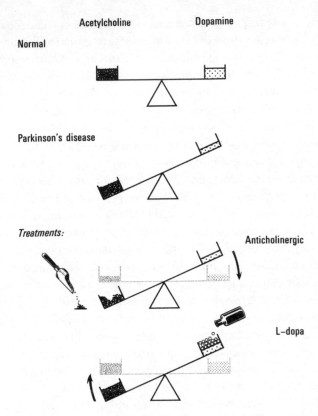

Fig. 5 The mutual interdependence of the chemical messenger dopamine and acetylcholine and how L-dopa and anticholinergic medicines can help to correct the imbalance.

balance between these two crucial neurotransmitters (Fig. 5). Although less effective than levodopa (to be discussed later), anticholinergic preparations are helpful when muscle stiffness and rigidity are dominant and they are still the first treatment prescribed for many patients. Among the unusual features and paradoxes of post-encephalitic parkinsonism is the fact that afflicted patients can tolerate very large doses of anticholinergic drugs without side-effects and with considerable benefit for many years. Anticholinergic drugs can also be given to patients with drug-induced parkinsonism when it is essential for their medical health to continue to take potent tranquillizers.

Undesirable effects are common because acetylcholine is the chief chemical messenger in the special part of the nervous system which controls the functions of digestion, heart rhythm, and glandular secretion. When accidental poisoning occurs the patient becomes hot, flushed, confused, and has defective near vision, adverse effects which have been pithily described as 'hot as a hare, dry as a bone, red as a beet, blind as a bat, and mad as a hatter'. Those who eat the berries of the deadly nightshade experience similar symptoms. Careful dose regulation prevents these problems, but the anticholinergic drugs should not be given to elderly men with enlargement of the prostate gland as an inability to pass urine may be provoked. They are also potentially dangerous in those suffering from glaucoma and, in the elderly, anticholinergic drugs may enhance confusion, accentuate forgetfulness, and simulate symptoms of mental illness. If, because of these unacceptable side-effects, it becomes necessary to stop anticholinergic medication this should be done gradually as abrupt cessation in a patient who has gained modest but useful benefit can cause marked physical deterioration. In brief, the benefits of anticholinergic drugs are, at best, modest; the possible side-effects and hazards, particularly in the elderly, are considerable. These drugs are still prescribed but caution is required.

Surgical treatments

The next phase in the development of effective treatments stems from James Parkinson's perspicacity. In his essay he mentioned a patient whose shaking improved when he had a stroke. This was later confirmed by others and formed the basis of neurosurgical treatment when it became possible to simulate this natural experiment. The aim was to suppress tremor without causing weakness of the limbs, and during the 1930s a number of surgical procedures were carried out on the pathways controlling voluntary movement in the brain and in the spinal cord. Early results were unpredictable and largely unsatisfactory: the patient often exchanged his tremor for weakness. By careful analysis of the bad as well as the encouraging results, Russell Meyers, an American surgeon, deduced that improved results could be achieved by dividing a small but critical bundle of nerve fibres within the brain called the ansa lenticularis. The safest way to accomplish this without damaging neighbouring vital structures involved a technique known as stereotactic surgery: a thin probe is delicately inserted into the brain through a hole in the skull. Accurate placement requires the co-operation of the alert patient so the procedure is performed under local anaesthetic with the patient lightly sedated.

As stereotactic techniques became more precise, sophisticated, and safe, so the scope, potential, and limitations of surgical treatments became clearer. The most impressive and enduring results were secured when the patient's main disability was severe, incapacitating tremor mainly occurring on one side of the body. In these circumstances the results could be spectacular. Generalized tremor necessitated bilateral operations and we learned that these were more hazardous. The beneficial effects on rigidity were less impressive and enduring and there was no improvement in brady-kinesia which was sometimes made worse. Frail, elderly patients with poor balance, speech disturbance, and predominant brady-kinesia fared very poorly. Increasing awareness of the indications for successful surgical treatment led, of course, to increasingly stringent selection criteria and gradually fewer operations were recommended. By 1967, only about one in ten patients were advised to have surgical treatment and today even fewer undergo such surgery. To some extent this swing away from brain surgery was a measure of the success of the recently introduced medicines. Now that we know the measure and limitations of these we can also see more clearly the indications for surgery. Physicians tend to be more conservative than surgeons and the notion of treating an illness by provoking further focal damage to the brain has always been difficult to accept. If a patient has a severe and incapacitating tremor on one side of the body, preferably the non-dominant side (left side in a right-handed person), with minimal bradykinesia, a good surgical result can be anticipated.

L-dopa (levodopa) treatment

The role of dopamine as a neurotransmitter in the brain and its deficiency in Parkinson's disease was described in a previous chapter. Dopamine is formed in the body from dopa, a relatively simple chemical—3,4-dihydroxyphenylalanine—which belongs to a group of substances called amino acids. These are made up of atoms of carbon, hydrogen, oxygen, and nitrogen, and are fundamental constituents of living matter. Dopa occurs naturally in many animals and plants and was first isolated in 1912 from the broad bean. One kilogram of these beans contains 25 grams of dopa and even higher concentrations occur in another leguminous plant, the cowhage (*Mucuna pruriens*, Plate VI), which grows throughout the tropical areas of America, India, and Africa. For many years it was recommended in India as an aphrodisiac and in Europe for curing worms. The immunity of many leguminous plants to attack from insects has been attributed to their high dopa content.

Levodopa or L-dopa is made in the body from another amino acid called tyrosine, which is present in protein-containing foods, but can also be made in our tissues from an essential dietary amino acid called phenylalanine. The rate of formation of L-dopa is strictly controlled by an enzyme called tyrosine hydroxylase (enzymes are proteins present in very small quantities in the body which regulate important chemical changes without themselves being used up during the reaction). Such is the accuracy of this controlling mechanism that an increase in dietary tyrosine will not augment the amount of available L-dopa. If this monitoring apparatus was not provided by nature, every time we ate a protein-rich meal, uncontrolled chemical changes would occur in our brains (Fig. 6). L-dopa is changed to the crucial neurotransmitter dopamine by the action of another enzyme. Fortunately for parkinsonian patients this second step is not rate-controlled and it is possible to increase the amount of dopamine in the brain by giving more L-dopa. When dopamine is given by mouth or by injection it is destroyed in the bloodstream so that it cannot be used to bolster the amounts needed in the parkinsonian brain.

Pioneer studies with L-dopa were carried out in the early 1960s by Birkmayer and Hornykiewicz in Vienna and Barbeau in Montreal. At that time, the world supplies of this hitherto ignored amino acid were very limited and only small doses for short periods could be given, but nevertheless startling, if ephemeral, improvement was observed in some patients. It was not until 1967

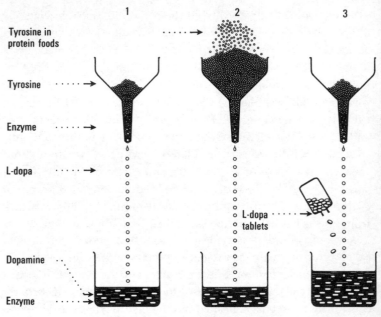

Fig. 6 Illustrating dopamine formation in the brain and how L-dopa treatment bypasses this.

when Cotzias in New York gave large amounts of L-dopa that the true potential of this form of treatment was realized. These early spectacular results were reported in medical journals, unleashing vociferous demands for L-dopa by doctors, patients, and relatives, and for a short time an international black-market flourished. Research both in the laboratory and the clinic thrived even more and a great deal is now known about L-dopa and its effects.

When L-dopa is taken by mouth it passes from the stomach into the small intestine where it is absorbed through the lining of the bowel wall into the bloodstream. This process takes time and is one of the reasons for the delayed action of L-dopa. Delay in emptying of the stomach can produce a further lag. This can be partly remedied by chewing the tablets and taking them with a glass of fruit juice. If L-dopa is taken with a large meal, absorption is delayed because other amino acids present in the food compete with L-dopa for absorption in the bowel. Thus, after an oral dose of L-dopa, two or three hours may elapse before maximum amounts appear in the blood, although small quantities are present after half an hour and some is still present after six hours. Absorbed L-dopa travels round the body in the bloodstream where much of it is changed into dopamine and destroyed in the kidney (to be excreted in the urine). At best, only about 10 per cent of the original dose taken by mouth reaches the brain intact. About 20 minutes is also required for L-dopa to cross the barrier between the bloodstream and the brain so that maximum brain levels are not achieved for some two and a half hours after taking L-dopa by mouth.

The enzyme which changes L-dopa to dopamine is called dopa-decarboxylase. As well as occurring in the brain it is present in large quantities in the blood vessels. It is this peripheral (outside the brain) destruction of L-dopa which is mainly responsible for the excessive wastage. When certain chemicals (called peripheral decarboxylase inhibitors) that could selectively prevent the action of the enzyme dopa-decarboxylase in the blood and thus allow a much greater portion of digested L-dopa to reach the brain were discovered, a further advance was made. Combinations of L-dopa with an appropriate amount of a peripheral decarboxylase inhibitor conveniently prepared in one pill or capsule is now the treatment of choice in Parkinson's disease. This valuable refinement of drug administration means that only about one-quarter of the amount of L-dopa is needed to produce the same benefits as before and, because there is a more rapid build-up of dosage and delivery to the brain, the onset of improvement usually takes place within an hour of taking the pill.

Two similar proprietary preparations are now widely available in the UK. Sinemet contains the inhibitor carbidopa and is made by Merck, Sharp & Dohme; Madopar, available throughout the world, but not in the USA, contains a different inhibitor called benserazide and is manufactured by Roche. Sinemet is now available in four forms: Sinemet 275 (250 mg of L-dopa and 50 mg of carbidopa), Sinemet 110 (100 mg of L-dopa and 10 mg carbidopa), Sinemet Plus (100 mg of L-dopa and 25 mg of carbidopa), and Sinemet LS (50 mg of L-dopa and 12.5 mg of carbidopa). All four are supplied as half-scored, oval tablets with appropriate distinctive marking. Madopar is marketed in equally convenient capsules of 62.5, 125, and 250 mg, each containing 50, 100, and 200 mg of L-dopa, respectively. A minority of patients with special problems may benefit from recently introduced controlled-release preparations of Sinemet and Madopar. These are usually given in combination with a standard preparation and require experienced supervision. There is also a dispersible liquid form of Madopar which is particularly useful for patients who have difficulty in swallowing. Even with combination treatment when the dosage can be built up rapidly, one or two weeks may elapse before a definite improvement is noticed, presumably because brain stores of dopamine are so low that many replenishing loads are required. If L-dopa is inadvertently and abruptly stopped, deterioration may continue for up to ten days. When treatment is resumed benefit recurs.

The benefits of L-dopa

Soon after starting treatment patients usually feel more alert, lively, and notice a facility of movement which they had almost forgotten. In mildly affected individuals, early in the course of their illness, the benefits may be so remarkable that all the symptoms and signs of their disease disappear and it may be impossible even for an experienced physician to diagnose the occult disease; in severely disabled individuals who have never been treated with L-dopa before and who have slowly become dependent upon others to feed, dress, and bathe, the benefit may be astonishing to patients and families alike (Fig. 7). Providing the diagnosis is correct, the majority of patients with Parkinson's disease gain useful benefit from L-dopa ranging from slight to spectacular. There is no particular clinical or laboratory test which will accurately predict the extent and nature of the response, but in general bradykinesia responds best, rigidity next, and tremor least and most slowly. Instability with a tendency to fall is the most refractory symptom of all and hardly ever responds well. In the early days of L-dopa therapy—and it will be recalled that most of the initial patients had advanced disease of long duration—the patients would often remark that the advent of L-dopa had given them back three or four years of life.

Most patients initially find that they can obtain a smooth response by taking their medication thrice daily after meals. As

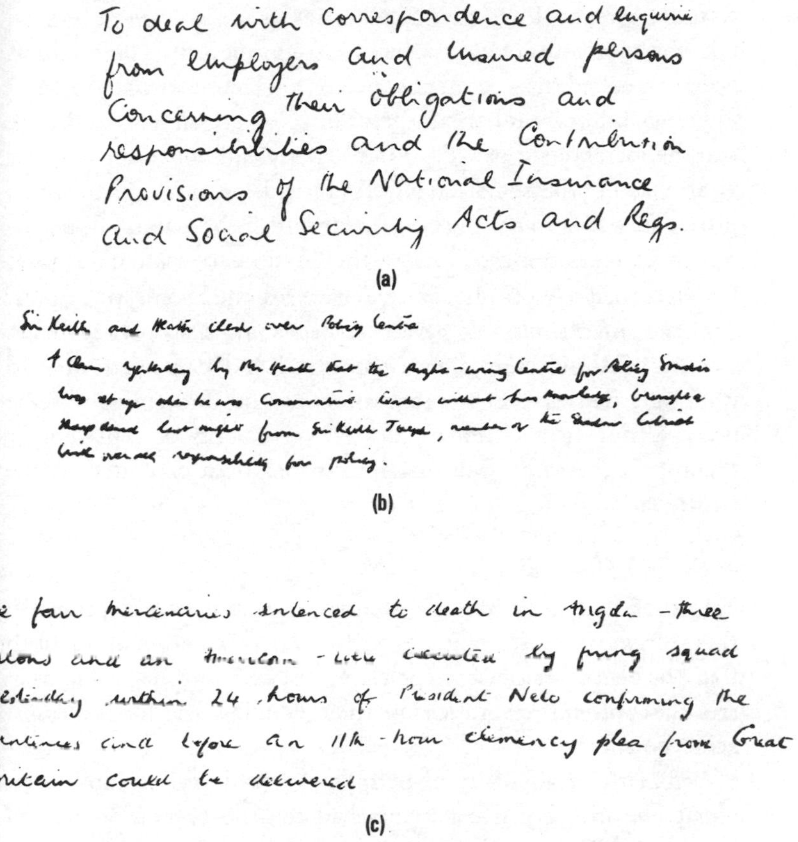

To deal with correspondence and enquiries
from employers and insured persons
concerning their obligations and
responsibilities and the contribution
provisions of the National Insurance
and Social Security Acts and Regs.

(a)

Sir Keith and Martin clash over Policy Centre

A claim yesterday by Mr Heath that the Right-wing Centre for Policy Studies was set up when he was Conservative leader without his knowledge, brought a sharp denial last night from Sir Keith Joseph, member of the Shadow Cabinet with overall responsibility for policy.

(b)

...e four mercenaries sentenced to death in Angola — three
...lons and an American — were executed by firing
squad
yesterday within 24 hours of President Neto confirming the
sentences and before an 11th-hour clemency plea from Great
Britain could be delivered

(c)

Fig. 7 Serial examples of a patient's handwriting (a) two years before the onset of Parkinson's disease, (b) first visit to hospital: increasingly small and illegible handwriting, (c) after six months of L-dopa treatment showing striking improvement in size and clarity.

time passes and treatment is continued, the duration of benefit from each dose appears to get less and the effects of an individual dose may wane after as little as one hour whereas previously a favourable response could be four to five hours in duration. The degree of benefit fortunately does not lessen to the same degree and by taking smaller doses more frequently it is often possible to restore some of the original improvement. Most patients shrewdly work this out before they consult their doctor and it is now commonplace to learn that small doses of medication have been taken at hourly intervals in order to preserve mobility. This curious change is called the 'on–off phenomenon'. The exact mechanism is unknown but it is probably largely due to progression of the disease and the metabolism of L-dopa in the body and not to tolerance or wearing-off of the beneficial effects of the drug. It is difficult to do justice in words to the overall benefit which thousands of parkinsonian patients can attribute to their L-dopa treatment. Typists have returned to work, housewives have resumed domestic responsibilities, precarious jobs have become secure, and, perhaps most striking of all, life expectancy is improved. L-dopa is not a cure and it cannot halt the slow progression of the underlying disease process, but it is a remarkably effective form of replacement therapy in the same way that insulin has been exploited in the treatment of sugar diabetes.

Side-effects of L-dopa

All drugs that work have side-effects; L-dopa is no exception. In this section, the disadvantages will be discussed at greater length than the benefits because, in practice, discussion of the problems of treatment often takes more time than rejoicing over the successful achievements.

Before the availability of peripheral decarboxylase inhibitors, about one in every five patients had to stop L-dopa because of intolerance. Nausea, vomiting, loss of appetite, a metallic taste in the mouth, and heartburn were common occurrences. These side-effects are not entirely due, as one might expect, to the effect of the medicine on the stomach, but occur as a result of stimulation of a group of nerve cells in the lower part of the brain known as the vomiting centre. These cells normally act as warning devices to prevent poisons entering the body and are continuously sampling the bloodstream so that toxins can be detected before they cross into the brain. Gradually building up the appropriate dose of L-dopa reduces the risk of this side-effect and administration after meals with an anti-sickness preparation such as domperidone (Motilium)—not yet available in the USA—is helpful and has greatly reduced the occurrence of this complication. When taking the combined preparations Sinemet or Madopar, smaller amounts of dopamine are present in the blood and consequently vomiting is less likely.

Other unwanted 'peripheral' effects of L-dopa, which have been reduced by peripheral decarboxylase inhibitors, are those due to the action of dopamine on the heart and blood-pressure. Dopamine, like its chemical relatives adrenalin and noradrenalin, has powerful stimulating effects on the blood-pressure and is now used to raise blood-pressure in circulatory failure in other patients. Paradoxically the blood-pressure may fall when L-dopa is given by mouth, and occasionally dizziness or fainting attacks can occur when the patient stands up suddenly. These effects also benefit from combined treatment and if the fainting tendency is persistent —tolerance often occurs without any specific treatment—the wearing of elastic stockings, an increased intake of salt, and the addition of a drug called fudrocortisone may be helpful.

Many patients are concerned whether it is safe to take other medicines with L-dopa. With two exceptions the answer is 'yes'. All the commonly prescribed medicines such as antibiotics, painkillers, travel sickness pills, hypnotics, local anaesthetics, and general anaesthetics can all be taken with confidence. Equally safe are vaccinations and alcohol in moderation. Similarly minor tranquillizers such as diazepam (Valium) and chlordiazepoxide (Librium) carry no hazard and the commonly prescribed antidepressants such as amytriptyline (Tryptizol), imipramine (Tofranil), and prothiaden (Dothiepin) can all be usefully combined with L-dopa. However, there is one particular group of antidepressants called monoamine oxidase inhibitors which must *never* be combined with L-dopa. These medicines, which include phenelzine (Nardil) and tranylcypromine (Parnate), are still widely prescribed for anxiety and depression and if unwittingly given to patients taking L-dopa, thumping headaches, palpitations, and potentially serious rises in blood-pressure may occur. At least three weeks should elapse after discontinuing these monoamine oxidase inhibitors before commencing L-dopa.

In the early days of L-dopa treatment some patients found that their condition deteriorated when they took vitamin supplements. This was because of large amounts of vitamin B_6 (pyridoxine) in these preparations. It has since been shown that whereas small amounts of pyridoxine are essential to assist the enzyme dopa-decarboxylase to convert dopa to dopamine, in the presence of very large doses of the vitamin the conversion to dopamine takes place too rapidly and consequently little reaches the brain.

Patients currently taking combined preparations with a peripheral decarboxylase inhibitor need not worry about this restriction as carbidopa and benserazide counteract this particular effect. Finally, it should be stressed that the major tranquillizers such as chlorpromazine (Largactil), thioridazine (Melleril), and haloperidol (Serenace) themselves produce parkinsonism and will aggravate pre-existing disabilities. Similarly prochlorperazine (Stemetil) and metoclopramide (Maxolon) for nausea should be avoided.

Mental changes always cause understandable anxiety. Most patients after commencing L-dopa feel more lively and seem to be more animated and alert. The ability to dream may return and refractory depression may be alleviated. Very occasionally, mild confusion occurs about an hour after each dose, but this is exceptional. When L-dopa first became available it predictably received irresponsible and sensational coverage. Newspaper head-lines such as 'sick old men chasing nurses' frightened many patients although admittedly it encouraged others to seek the drug. Although an increased libido occasionally occurs this is no more than would be expected following recovery from a chronic, debilitating illness and would not be construed as an undesirable side-effect. However, a few patients develop more serious reactions which can include intense restlessness, intolerable anxiety, un-realistic grandiose ideas, or paranoid feelings that their nearest relatives are trying to harm them in some way. Mild confusional states are particularly likely in the elderly who already may have some degree of forgetfulness. Delirium with disorientation may be provoked. Particular attention should be drawn to frightening nightmares and vivid visual hallucinations. The latter are more common towards the evening when the patient may see imaginary animals or human figures or experience the intense sensation that another person is close behind him. All these problems are reversible when L-dopa is reduced or, if necessary, stopped.

The most common complication of long-term L-dopa treatment

is the development of abnormal involuntary movements called dyskinesias. These are thought to arise from degenerating nerve cells which are in a state of hyperexcitability and are 'supersensitive' to neurotransmitters such as dopamine. When the initial dose of L-dopa is high, dyskinesias may appear during the first year of treatment, but they usually become troublesome after two or three years of medication. Usually first observed by friends and relatives rather than the patient, fidgetiness, twitching of the lips and face, eyebrow raising, grimacing, tongue protrusion, or curling of the toes may appear from time to time. These additional movements are more evident when the patient is mobile and when he is obtaining maximum benefit from treatment. While the face and mouth are most commonly affected, writhing, jerky movements of the arms and neck and uncontrollable kicking or paddling movements of the legs may develop; rapid sighs or panting may disturb the rhythm of breathing. These movements are called interdose dyskinesias because they are worst when L-dopa concentration in the blood is high. Movements usually begin about half an hour after each dose of L dopa and may persist for up to two or three hours. In some people two discrete attacks of severe dyskinesia (onset and end-of-dose) occur between each dose. While great variability of pattern occurs, the movements are usually more severe on the side initially affected with Parkinson's disease and it is possible at certain times of the day for one half of the body to be stiff and immobile while the other is affected by involuntary movements. Dyskinesias always improve when the dose of L-dopa is reduced, but at the expense of increasing slowness, stiffness, and tremor. A commonsense compromise has to be established for each individual and this rarely constitutes a problem when the patient and his family have experienced the two extremes. For example, one builder opted for a higher mid-week dose as he was prepared to accept more involuntary movements in exchange for mobility at work, then took a smaller dose at the weekends so that his family should not be distressed by seeing the unwanted movements.

Painful spasms and cramps affecting the feet particularly on awakening in the morning are another common problem. The foot tends to turn inwards involuntarily with clawing of the toes, except for the big toe which may be lifted up. Stamping or stretching the muscles helps, but the spasms usually clear spontaneously within half an hour after the first dose of L-dopa. Occasionally, spasms of the jaw occur making chewing and talking difficult. Although these distressing cramps occasionally occur in patients not taking medication, they seem very much more common when L-dopa has been taken for many years.

Although this list of possible drawbacks sounds rather discouraging there can be no doubt whatsoever that L-dopa remains the most effective treatment for Parkinson's disease and when the dose and timing have been tailor-made according to an individual's requirements a great deal of improvement can be expected. The decision of when to start L-dopa requires careful consideration, particularly if the illness is very mild. At present, most doctors prefer to withhold L-dopa until there is definite evidence that disabilities are beginning to affect everyday activities. This policy is based on the notion that medication has a finite period of maximal usefulness—unfortunately termed the 'honeymoon period'—and that side-effects are more likely to appear when the drug has been used in high doses. Another approach is to begin L-dopa as soon as the diagnosis has been established, but keeping the total daily dose at a low level, leaving something in reserve for the years ahead. In this manner some immediate benefit can be obtained with fewer complications.

Other medicines

Amantadine

Amantadine (Symmetrel) was originally used to protect patients from certain virus infections such as influenza and shingles. In 1968, a lady with Parkinson's disease who began to take amantadine reported to her doctor that she felt more mobile. This original observation prompted careful trials in several specialist centres which confirmed the patient's opinion. Improvement was not spectacular, but modest improvement in tremor, rigidity, and bradykinesia unquestionably occurred in some patients, although unfortunately not all, and the benefits seem to wane after a few months. It is still a mystery how amantadine works, but it has been suggested that it might increase the release of dopamine from nerve cells and possibly prevent its re-storage. Unwanted effects include visual hallucinations, delirium, nausea, dry mouth, and blurred vision. Rarely, swelling of the ankles with a purplish, marbled discoloration of the shins develops called livedo reticularis. Fortunately, all these complications disappear when the drug is withdrawn. Overall, amantadine is slightly more potent than anticholinergic medications, although the benefits do not last as long, and it can be usefully combined with L-dopa in some patients.

Bromocriptine

Bromocriptine (Parlodel) was originally synthesized to prevent the formation of milk in women who elected not to breast-feed their infants. It is derived from an alkaloid called ergot which is obtained from a rye fungus which in the past, when it contaminated millers' flour, caused epidemics of gangrene, convulsions, and insanity—the so-called St Anthony's fire. Ergot compounds which have the property of causing certain muscles to contract have been used in medicine for many years to treat migraine and to aid in the expulsion of the afterbirth following delivery of a baby. Bromocriptine has been found to mimic the effects of dopamine in the brain by stimulating the dopamine receptors on nerve cells. It was therefore soon tried in the treatment of Parkinson's disease and was shown to have powerful antiparkinsonian effects when given in relatively large doses. Although it is more potent than the anticholinergic preparations or amantadine its usefulness in the treatment of Parkinson's disease seems to be rather limited. It has been given to patients who, despite taking maximum amounts of L-dopa, are slowly losing ground and partial substitution of L-dopa by bromocriptine may help a few patients. However, our experience with bromocriptine in this situation—namely when optimum benefit has been squeezed out of L-dopa—has been disappointing. It is possible that bromocriptine could be given to newly diagnosed patients so that L-dopa can be held in reserve, perhaps delaying the onset of complications such as dyskinesias and oscillations in performance. It has also been suggested that combined low-dose L-dopa and bromocriptine from the start of treatment may offer certain advantages. Comparative trials are under way, but it will be evident from a disease which runs a course of several decades that it may take years before an answer emerges. Like all potent medicines, side-effects occur and these include vomiting, nausea, lethargy, and muzzy headaches—all very similar to L-dopa but tending to occur more frequently—and also certain psychiatric upsets. These include confusion, agitation, depression, excitability, and particularly intense and vivid visual hallucinations which may persist for several weeks after bromocriptine is withdrawn. This is not surprising because the chemical structure of bromocriptine is similar to that of the psychedelic drug lysergic acid. The taking of bromocriptine by patients already using L-dopa may cause more involuntary movements and it may then be difficult to know which medicine should be reduced or withdrawn. Bromocriptine is a member of a family of drugs called dopamine agonists which work by stimulating dopamine receptors. Other members of this group are apomorphine, pergolide, and lisuride. Such drugs may be useful adjuncts to L-dopa in the management of certain carefully selected problems, but experienced supervision is required.

Deprenyl

Deprenyl (Eldepryl) was synthesized in Hungary and in the 1960s it was reported to possess 'psychic energizing' properties. It belongs to a class of drugs already mentioned called monoamine oxidase inhibitors, useful in the treatment of certain depressive illnesses. Monoamine oxidase is an enzyme present in many parts of the body including the brain, blood vessels, liver, and other organs, and is responsible for mopping up excessive amounts of monoamines such as adrenalin, noradrenalin, and also dopamine. This protective system can be blocked by monoamine oxidase inhibitors. The long established 'conventional' monoamine oxidase inhibitors, as previously discussed, must never be taken with L-dopa or foodstuffs such as cheese, Marmite, Chianti wine, or pickled herrings, and patients are always issued with a card telling them the foods they must avoid. If the controlling enzyme is inactivated, these foodstuffs can generate excessive quantities of noradrenalin, provoking headache, palpitations, and potentially serious increases in blood-pressure. Deprenyl possesses the extraordinary quality of selectivity, blocking only the enzyme which destroys dopamine and allowing the normal degradation of other monoamines to continue. Deprenyl is therefore free of these restricting 'cheese effects' yet it is able to increase dopamine in the brain by preventing its normal breakdown within nerve cells and in the gaps between the nerve fibres. As a result it can be used safely with L-dopa or any of its combinations and dietary restrictions are unnecessary.

When given alone deprenyl has negligible effects on the disabilities of Parkinson's disease, but it can enhance the action of small doses of L-dopa. More importantly, the addition of deprenyl may smoothe out the mild 'on–off' effects of L-dopa. It has the advantage that it is easy to use, a single morning dose of 10 mg (or two doses, 5 mg at breakfast and 5 mg at lunch) is required and its unwanted side-effects are singularly few. It seems that deprenyl has a useful, if limited, adjuvant role in the treatment of Parkinson's disease.

It was recently suggested on theoretical speculation that deprenyl might have a beneficial effect on Parkinson's disease by slowing down the underlying illness and possibly giving protection against suspected environmental toxins. Naturally such a claim provoked great interest and long-term trials were initiated to try and confirm or refute this proposal. The presently available 'facts' are insufficient to justify deprenyl for all parkinsonian patients. In the USA, a multicentred trial is laboriously comparing deprenyl, vitamin E, and placebo in hitherto untreated patients. In the UK, a trial is underway comparing standard L-dopa therapy with L-dopa plus deprenyl, or bromocriptine. Experience dictates patience and caution lest unjustified conclusions are drawn; it is difficult to accept this sober advice when you are disabled, but nevertheless necessary. Analysis of initial results of these trials is encouraging: deprenyl given early in the course of the illness before L-dopa is given may slow down but not stop the progress of the illness.

We do not have as yet—despite many trials—effective medical treatments to help disturbances of balance and 'freezing' of gait, when the patient has difficulty in initiating walking or turning in confined spaces. As these upsets are not constant and the motor system can work for some of the time, it should prove possible to correct when we understand more about the working of the human 'gear box'. For the present, physiotherapy techniques such as using visual landmarks and auditory reinforcement offer the best hope of improvement.

Reference has already been made to fluctuations or oscillations in performance and motor disabilities experienced by some patients who have taken L-dopa with benefit for several years. The pattern of such swings from incapacity to well nigh normality varies greatly from patient to patient. For example, some feel particularly mobile and well on awakening and can defer the first dose of medication for several hours; others may be so stiff and immobile at dawn that they will set their alarm clocks in order to take medication an hour before arising. Some feel their best in the latter third of the day while others feel weary and jaded. For these, judicious adjustments to the timing and size of doses may be helpful; the regimen has to be tailored to individual requirements. Avoiding meals containing large amounts of protein, which can compete with L-dopa for absorption in the gut and at the blood-brain barrier, may help others. For some, the addition of deprenyl, bromocriptine, or long-acting L-dopa preparations may iron out some of these undulations.

At one time 'drug holidays' were recommended. It was proposed that stopping all medications for several days allowed the receptors to regain full responsiveness when drugs were re-introduced. The claim could not be confirmed as the technique proved to be very dangerous for certain patients. This strategy is no longer advised.

However, there is a small group of patients whose fluctuations are so extreme and incapacitating and resistant to all the above strategies (their illness usually begins at a younger age) who require special attention. We know that constant intravenous infusions of L-dopa or dopamine agonists such as lisuride can control most of the oscillations and keep such individuals 'on' for much longer periods. Unfortunately, it is not practical to do this for long periods. It is possible, however, to give apomorphine (a drug which stimulates dopamine receptors and which occurs in nature, see Plate VII) by subcutaneous injection to produce the same benefit—rather like giving insulin to a diabetic patient. Apomorphine may be given by repeated injection just before a patient knows that he is about to go 'off'; for more severe fluctuations a continuous subcutaneous infusion controlled by an electronic pump may be required. It is usually necessary to admit patients to hospital for a short period so that their individual requirements can be determined. This is a new technique and we still have much to learn about it.

Summary

Although this section concerning medical treatments has been based upon questions often asked by patients and their families, we are conscious that it is somewhat indigestible. It does however emphasize the continuing need for careful discussion between patient and doctor. This is of course valuable in all illnesses, but it is essential in the management of Parkinson's disease. An adequate explanation of symptoms, the mechanism of drug actions, and what can be reasonably expected from treatment is a very personal matter and may require repeated discussion. Complicated drug combinations consisting of one or more medicines will not be pursued unless explanation has been clear and comprehensible. Only in this way can abortive visits to a series of hospital specialists in search of an elusive panacea be prevented. In this matter, the advice of the first century physician Celsus cannot be improved — 'you should prefer a physician who is your friend to a stranger if their knowledge is equal'.

5. How to live with Parkinson's disease

A retired general who had fought his Parkinson's disease with courage, ingenuity, and humour insisted on starting the day with a swim. As he entered his eighties and his disabilities slowly increased, swimming several lengths was slowly reduced to limited exercises at the shallow end. On hearing this news his doctor foolishly attempted to comfort him by saying that many men of his years free of illness had long given up all forms of exercise. There was an icy pause, the general twitched his moustache and mischievously remarked 'Yes, but they are civilians'.

It has been our privilege to talk to many patients with Parkinson's disease and we have learned that of all the actions that patients can take to help themselves, acquiring a determined, positive attitude of mind to combat illness is by far the most important and effective. A prolonged campaign against an ever-present enemy is a difficult task. Those who accept the challenge to their independence and exercise every possible stratagem against invalidism invariably do better than those who deny their illness or who needlessly become dependent upon others.

Successfully living with the illness often depends upon relatively simple adjustments to one's life style. For example, a deliberate decision must be made to allocate adequate time to dressing, preparing for work, and travelling. Most of these are commonsense decisions, but we should like to consider certain specific problems.

Diet

Try to keep slim and avoid obesity; you should not add to your disabilities by carrying needless weight. There are no specific food items to be avoided except for those containing too many calories. For example, you need not alter your intake of beer, wine, and spirits providing this is modest and you are not overweight. If you are receiving levodopa therapy and experiencing marked fluctuations in performance (the on–off effect) a reduction in the amount of dietary protein may be advisable. For most people the easiest way to do this is to severely restrict protein at breakfast and lunch and then eat a normal dinner late in the day. Protein is present in all types of meat, dairy products, and nuts. If constipation is troublesome eat more fresh fruit, vegetables, and roughage such as bran.

Physical activity, exercises, and physiotherapy

A general rule is to be as active as the condition permits without provoking undue fatigue. Fears that exhaustion or weariness will cause setbacks or deterioration are absolutely groundless. Frequent short bursts of physical activity are preferable to irregular marathons. Whatever the duration or severity of the malady it is essential to remain active and to persist with regular exercise in keeping with one's strength and mobility. Those who were previously unathletic and sedentary may require a great deal of encouragement from relatives and friends and a minority must be firmly persuaded to include more exercise in their daily routine. However, care must be taken when first embarking on a new form of exercise. For example, some patients have described difficulties when swimming and maintaining their balance in water. The exact nature of the exercise or sport matters little providing it is enjoyable and easily organized. It is essential to maintain normal posture, balance, and muscle tone because in the absence of appropriate movement muscles stiffen and joints become restricted and painful.

For those who are incapacitated despite appropriate treatments probably the most beneficial activity is an unhurried walk taken at a set time in the company of a sympathetic companion. Comfortable shoes are important and the route can be chosen to avoid crowds, traffic, and arduous hills. Gentle keep-fit exercises at home for ten minutes, four times a day are helpful and the main joints should be put through a full range of movement several times in order to stretch rigid muscles. Avoid strenuous exercises such as press-ups or toe-squats and concentrate on rhythmical, easily accomplished movements such as swinging the arms.

Breathing exercises consisting of deep inspirations with maximum chest expansion will stretch the chest wall and help carry oxygen to poorly aerated parts of the lung. Relaxation techniques can be of inestimable value in helping to allay tension. Books, tapes, and classes are widely available and some hospitals run yoga classes. Grimacing and making faces in front of the mirror counters immobility of facial muscles. When walking, endeavour to prevent the length of the stride diminishing. This can be accomplished at home by making marks on the floor and ensuring that these are cleared. Postural stooping can be combated by exercises with the back in contact with the wall. The general aim is to maintain rhythm and co-ordination in a relaxed manner.

Each patient has an individual problem and it is here that the advice of a physiotherapist can be particularly helpful. Unlike patients who have had a stroke, parkinsonians are not paralysed and their muscle strength is usually normal. The essential difficulty is in initiating quick movements and in sustaining regular actions over a period of time. The mechanism which underlies the execution of normal movement can be strengthened by stimulation from the eyes, speech, and touch in the following manner. Careful attention to lines on the carpet or cracks in the paving stones can often overcome freezing attacks and facilitate the initiation and maintenance of a fluent, rhythmical stride. Listening to or humming marching music with a clear-cut rhythm, the sound of a ticking metronome, or the stimulus of a regularly shifting white handkerchief from one hand to the other when walking are tricks which have proved useful to some of our patients. This technique of so-called 'sensory reinforcement' can also be used to great effect with group classes when the instructor tries to reinforce movement and gesture by accompanying physical exercise with clear-cut, decisive, rhythmical instructions. Exercises of this kind are preferably performed on a daily basis at home and are far more valuable than occasional sporadic hospital visits to physiotherapy departments. Music therapy may also improve the melody of body movements and the purchase of a portable, personal stereo can be of great use provided the music is chosen judiciously.

The exact combination of exercises must of course be selected according to an individual's needs, but the following suggestions can usually be practised at home and will help in overcoming frustrating difficulties.

Rising from a chair

Wriggle towards the edge of the seat and place the heels as far back under the chair as possible. Lean well forwards from the hips so that the centre of gravity is directly above the feet and gently rise to the standing position. If necessary, push down on the sides of the chair to achieve a smooth movement.

Walking

Normally the heel strikes the ground first, followed by the toes. In Parkinson's disease there is a tendency for this pattern to be reversed so that the toes touch the ground first, leading to a stooped posture and instability. Therefore, when walking is difficult, deliberately place the heel first and reinforce this by repeating 'heel first' rhythmically with each stride. If the balance is affected when turning, try to walk in a semi-circle rather than twist round on the spot.

Freezing

If your feet seem to be rooted to the ground, slowly stand up as straight as possible. Start walking slowly and deliberately lift one leg, bending the hip and knee, and place it in front. Another technique is to take a small step backwards before moving forward, to initiate rhythmical movement. Rocking gently from one foot to the other may liberate walking movements; some patients find that if they make a sideways step like a crab they may then be able to walk off in a normal manner. Use visual cues to maximum advantage, deliberately stepping over cracks in paving stones or patterns in the carpet. If walking with a companion they can often assist by placing their foot in front of yours and commanding you to step over the obstacle. Instruct your family never to attempt to pull you as this increases your difficulty, causes freezing to be more stubborn, and may cause you to fall. When the automatic reflexes of walking and balance are impaired, great concentration is required—rather like an actor performing on the stage—to compensate for them.

Turning in bed

When climbing into bed, first sit on the edge at the right position so that on lying down the head is comfortably placed on the pillow. If you find difficulty in turning when on your back, bend the hips and knees so the feet are flat, tuck both legs to the chosen side, then swing both arms forward towards the same side, gripping the edge of the bed and thereby turning. Alternatively, sit up first and then re-position.

Posture

A tendency to stoop can be combated by grasping both hands behind the back and bracing the shoulders back firmly several times a day and, as previously mentioned, exercises against a wall are helpful.

Speech exercises

Advice from a speech therapist should be sought as soon as speech difficulties occur. If this is impossible, a tape of speech exercises is available through the Parkinson's Disease Society of the United Kingdom. If the voice is indistinct, practice reading aloud in front of the mirror, enunciating as clearly as possible and exaggerating the syllables like a ham actor. Such deliberate articulations can be of great help when the voice is tired or difficult to hear. Recitation in time to a slow, fixed beat is a similar exercise and it is important to breathe deeply at regular intervals. Speaking into a tape recorder may give you some idea of the difficulties experienced by others when they say that your speech is indistinct and this technique can also be used to monitor improvement. Exceptionally, the defect of speech is a very poor volume and here amplifiers for use on the telephone may be extremely valuable, particularly for those living alone.

Specific problems

Constipation

Parkinson's disease itself causes constipation by slowing down movements of the bowel and upsetting the control of the muscles of defecation. Drug treatment may also make the problem worse, particularly the anticholinergic drugs [benzhexol (Artane) and orphenadrine (Disipal)] and some pain-killers such as codeine. Take plenty of exercise, fluid with meals, and make sure the diet contains adequate fibre from vegetables, fruit, bran-containing breakfast cereals, and wholemeal bread. A soft bowel action two or three times a week is quite reasonable. Bulk laxatives such as Normacol, Fybogel, or Celevac are to be preferred but sometimes irritant laxatives such as Dulcolax or Dorbanex are needed. Lactulose (Duphalac) and docusate sodium (Dioctyl) may be helpful if the stool is very hard. Occasionally, severe constipation may require weekly suppositories or even enemas.

Dribbling of saliva from the mouth

This occurs because the tongue and throat muscles are not working efficiently and the head may be slightly bent forward allowing saliva to escape from the mouth. Exercises to improve facial muscle function and breathing may be helpful. Thick, tacky saliva accumulating at the back of the throat can be dispelled by a blackcurrant drink or honey topped up with hot water. Drugs such as anticholinergics which can dry up saliva can sometimes help but often lead to an equally intolerable dry mouth. In severe cases X-ray treatment to the salivary glands may be considered.

Insomnia

It is extremely important to try to obtain a restful night's sleep as this invariably improves function the following day. Difficulty turning, and getting in and out of bed, painful cramps, the need to repeatedly visit the lavatory, and vivid nightmares can all be problems on occasions. Before retiring, empty your bladder, take a warm bath or shower, a milky drink, and make sure your bed is warm and comfortable. A peaceful short walk before bed-time can also encourage relaxation. Avoid coffee, tea, or excess alcohol in the

evening; sleeping pills may occasionally be necessary, but often a
nocturnal dose of levodopa is even more effective.

Bladder problems

A need to go frequently and urgently to the lavatory to pass urine
can be a symptom of Parkinson's disease. In elderly, infirm men,
prostate trouble is also common, leading to urinary hesitancy and a
poor stream. This can be made worse by anticholinergic drugs
(Artane, Disipal, Kemadrin). Bladder infections (cystitis) can also
occur, particularly in women, causing frequency of urination,
scalding pain on passing water, and cloudy, offensive urine.
Bladder symptoms should always be reported promptly to the
family doctor who may then advise a specialist opinion.

Sexual difficulties

Most patients with Parkinson's disease have no trouble making
love but a few lose their sexual desire and some men become
impotent. Emotional factors or physical fatigue may be contribu-
tory. Occasionally, levodopa may actually increase libido. Assuming a recumbent posture underneath your partner may reduce
fatigue and pain. A consultation with your doctor should be
arranged to discuss these problems.

Aids to daily living

Intelligent application of mechanical aids can make the difference
between full independence and reliance upon relatives, neigh-
bours, and district nurses. Occupational therapists are particularly
well-informed about the possibilities and they usually prefer to
visit a patient's home to assess individual needs. Local social
services departments and the Disabled Living Foundation are also
useful sources of practical information and if there is any difficulty
in obtaining apparatus the Parkinson's Disease Society should be
contacted. Difficulty in securing shoelaces and in buttoning of
blouses and shirts occur when fingers are less dexterous and can
usually be circumvented by the use of zips, Velcro adhesive patches
sewn onto clothing, shoe horns, and slip-on shoes with elastic
fastenings. Clumsiness in holding cutlery can often be helped by

enlarging the handles of knives and forks with rubber foam secured with tape. For the more disabled, plates with raised edges, two-handled and non-spill cups, and suction egg cups are other simple but useful items of domestic equipment. If tremor is severe, drinking straws preserve independence and electric can openers, jar openers, and tap turners can also be helpful. Strategically placed bath rails and secure rubber mats facilitate getting in and out of the bath when slowness of movement and poor balance are incapacitating. Bath seats can be fitted on top or inside the bath so that the patient is able to slowly lower himself. A shower rather than a bath may be safer. A padded, elevated lavatory seat with appropriately placed hand rails can make a crucial difference. With respect to choice of furniture, deep upholstered chairs can be a great nuisance and should be avoided; straight-backed chairs with firm seats and reliable armrests are much to be preferred. Attention to home safety with fire guards for open fires, good lighting, comfortable footwear, and electric kettles is important.

The earlier models of spring-loaded ejection seats were rarely satisfactory because of the rapidity of action, but more recently introduced models with controlled elevation should be considered for the badly handicapped. Mechanically controlled beds which permit head elevation and turning can also be obtained, but most people find that a duvet, silk, or satin sheets and a rope ladder or monkey pole are all that is needed. Adjustable reading stands come in handy when books are awkward to hold and a felt-tipped pen and lined notepaper should be tried if handwriting becomes difficult. A walking stick or frame with wheels gives valuable security during freezing episodes and reduces the risk of falling, but in the open most patients prefer to walk without mechanical assistance. There are many useful aids for the kitchen, some of which are extremely simple. For example, it is more convenient and safer to cook vegetables in a wire basket which can then be removed, leaving the water to cool before pouring it away. For garden enthusiasts, specially designed tools are available which avoid the need to bend.

6. The future

When the patient and his family have come to grips with the illness, understood the potential and the limitations of current treatments, and have made the necessary adjustments to living with a chronic malady, they often ask about the implications of current scientific research and possible future developments. To attempt to summarize the flood of published scientific papers which have been largely stimulated by the successful evolution of levodopa would prove an impossible physical task. To consider the possible implications would require exceptional clairvoyance. Scientific as well as political and economic history teaches us that the experts are easily provoked into prediction, but are rarely found to be correct. For example, would a well-informed neurologist of the 1930s confidently anticipate that a common crippling disease of childhood, poliomyelitis, would completely disappear within his professional span of years? Would a neurologist of the 1950s think it possible that an effective medical treatment would become available for a degenerative disorder such as parkinsonism which could put a patient three years back in the course of his illness? An authoritative text-book of the time nihilistically commented that to expect truly useful treatments for such a disorder was akin to acquiring the very elixir of life. Such notions, as absurd as safely placing a man on the moon, could not be confidently anticipated by a sane and reasonable man. Yet we do live in an extraordinary world where science fiction fantasies have become incontrovertible scientific achievements. If, therefore, generous concession is made by the reader for present ignorance, fallibility, and almost total unpredictability a few armchair speculations on the way ahead might be cautiously considered.

For example, consider current developments in imaging techniques. Using a method called magnetic resonance imaging (MRI), it is now possible to measure the size and shape of structures deep in the brain, such as the substantia nigra, without discomfort or hazard to the patient (Plate VIII). Using a different technique called position emission tomography (PET) the amount of dopamine in the basal ganglia can now be estimated with considerable accuracy (Plate IX). Hitherto, information of this kind would only be obtained at post-mortem examination. We have entered a new era of mapping the brain during life. The possibilities of advancing our understanding of the brain in both health and disease are now boundless.

Clearly, a great deal has still to be learned about the neurotransmitter dopamine. What are the factors which determine formation, storage, and release of dopamine, and the nature of the feedback control mechanisms normally employed by the brain? The dopamine gold seam has yet to be completely exhausted, yet many scientists are coming to the opinion that we may have been unduly preoccupied with dopamine because its exploitation has been so immediately rewarding and because technically it has been relatively easy to study. We are increasingly aware of our ignorance concerning other known or possible transmitter substances and their complex interactions. For example, little is known to date about the interplay between the neurotransmitters dopamine and acetylcholine and even less is known about a substance called gamma-aminobutyric acid. In the last decade, the number of known chemical neurotransmitters in the brain has increased considerably with the recognition that a number of hormones occur in nerve cells. These substances—neuropeptides—could well act as important neurotransmitters. The list now exceeds forty but only a few have been adequately studied. It is quite possible that there are other critical substances and systems within our brains which to research workers are still as remote as the rings of Saturn. If each system can modulate the activity of the others by complex patterns of excitation and inhibition it may be necessary to invoke the assistance of advanced computer technology before we can even begin to understand the normal control of movement and its dissolution by disease.

Consider for a moment the nature and extraordinary variability of almost all the symptoms of Parkinson's disease. Relatives are often baffled by the surprising manner in which a disabled patient can rise to the occasion and put on an impeccable physical performance when attending hospital yet be completely unable to muster a comparable effort when at home. Tremor may wax and wane with baffling fickleness within the space of seconds; the normal resting posture can be disturbed by gross, incapacitating shaking. Equally dramatic and puzzling are the violent swings of neural control that have been dubbed 'on–off' oscillations; one moment the patient is able to walk gracefully to be followed within seconds by almost complete immobility. To these marked variations we must include freezing or being rooted to the ground after walking smoothly and the stranger paradoxes when the stiff rigid state can be dramatically relieved by an intense physical shock or emotional upset. Evidently the system—no matter how complex —between will and movement is always intact, but it is not continuously working or in gear. What then are the factors which determine and control the availability of motor systems? Is it fired by critical concentrations of neurotransmitter substances or does the mystery lie in fluctuating but crucial sensitivity of fields of specific receptors? If so, what are the biochemical mechanisms which subserve sensitivity and response? If, as in paralysis following a stroke, there was a gross structural disruption of the nervous system there would be little prospect of truly effective treatment, but as there is no paralysis in Parkinson's disease surely the puzzle of intermittent control should be soluble.

Consider, for example, the management of on–off oscillations. When these strange fluctuations were first initially recognized (around 1969) we were powerless to help such patients. Intensive research has now made available a variety of strategies—slow-release preparations of levodopa, selective drugs such as deprenyl which slow down the destruction of dopamine, dietary adjustments, and, very recently, the use of subcutaneous administration of apomorphine—to help many patients.

Turning to the field of drug action or pharmacology, all the auguries suggest that in the predictable future more refined and specific chemical agents will be available for trial. For example, the provocation of drug-induced dyskinesias, which is the most common factor limiting the amounts of L-dopa that can be comfortably taken, should be subject to finer control. Dyskinesias are generally attributed to differing states of sensitivity in different groups of receptors. Should it not be possible to find a safe and specific receptor-blocking drug which will only inhibit the systems responsible for dyskinesia and thereby allow more L-dopa to be taken without side-effects? Specificity of drug responses appear to depend on the lock and key principle. Only the exact fitting, that is the precise molecular structure, will act upon the appropriate receptor to unlock the desirable response. The chemical structure of deprenyl (selegiline) closely resembles that of a well-known drug called amphetamine and yet a relatively slight change in molecular structure confers a specific and desirable selective effect in blocking the destruction of dopamine in the brain. It is too defeatist to state blandly that new drugs simply bring new problems. The fact that serious sensitivity reactions may rarely occur after penicillin fortunately did not discourage its development and the subsequent search for more effective and safer antibiotics.

Turning to an entirely different area of research, recent studies into two animal and two uncommon human 'degenerative' brain diseases have provided evidence of a new concept in the cause of neurological disease. Scrapie affects sheep and goats and the mink may develop a curious brain disease well known to veterinary specialists. The two human illnesses are called Jakob–Creuzfeldt disease and Kuru. The cause of the former is thought to be an extremely small particle or virus-like agent which can pass through the finest of filters and which has a long incubation period. Kuru occurs among the Fore people of the eastern highlands of Papua New Guinea and literally means to shake from fever or cold. Epidemiological studies have revealed a curious distribution. The disease usually occurs in women and in children of both sexes. It now seems fairly firmly established that transmission of the illness occurs as a consequence of cannibalism during ceremonial rituals of mourning for the deceased. The shaking illness is slowly progressive and post-mortem findings include diffuse degenerative changes most consistently involving the cerebrum, the cerebellum, and the basal ganglia. All four diseases can be experimentally transmitted to animals by inoculations of affected brain material. After a long incubation period which may extend over years, when the features of the disease eventually appear, the course of the illness is progressive and relentless. It is still unknown whether these diseases are related and whether genetic susceptibility is an important factor. The properties of the transmissible particle remain extremely difficult to work out; but the concept of 'slow' infections in the nervous system of man and animals is now firmly established. Parkinson's disease, which is of course a much more common malady, has been intensively studied in a similar manner, but so far attempts to transmit the illness to laboratory animals have been disappointingly unsuccessful. Despite these setbacks, this new notion of an infectious agent which can remain symptomless in the body for many years before declaring itself will continue to be regarded with suspicion and will remain a challenge to further research.

The most exciting, controversial, and still unresolved development in the search for a remedy for Parkinson's disease concerns brain implant operations. The first experimental attempts to graft brain from one animal to another stems back to 1890, but it was not until 1979 that scientists demonstrated that rat fetal substantia nigra could be successfully grafted to a mature rat. Furthermore, the graft could correct the consequences of previously imposed damage to the rat's motor system.

After these results were confirmed it was not too long before brain implant operations were performed in parkinsonian patients. The first operations utilized the patient's own adrenal gland which contains dopamine-producing cells. Later, after considerable ethical and moral discussions, human fetal substantia nigra was used. All these operations must be considered to be no more than tentative experimental explorations far removed from the realities of practical effective treatments. We have much to learn about the basic biological mechanisms which determine whether a graft will survive and function in man. Hopefully, a new era of treatment has begun but the results so far counsel caution and patience: there is still much to be done.

Summary

Intensive research continues into possible causes of Parkinson's disease and there is no shortage of theories to confirm or refute:

healthy controversy reigns. It seemed at one time that hereditary factors had been firmly excluded and that attention should be exclusively directed to environmental factors such as chemicals, toxins, and pollutants. Certainly this seemed to be the lesson of the MPTP discoveries. However, it has recently been proposed that this is too simple an interpretation and that hereditary factors should not be totally discounted. Is it possible that genetical factors might influence an individual's susceptibility to one or more environmental factors? A new discipline—so-called ecogenetics—has arisen and is now receiving intensive study.

Perhaps all our current theories will prove to be wrong. Readers will recall the celebrated Father Brown detective stories. The sleuth had an axiom: the reason why we do not know the answer is because we do not know the right question to ask.

A few of the present fashionable speculations about the nature of Parkinson's disease and its treatment have been discussed here in a superficial manner. Such is the nature of research that it is likely that all these theories will not survive the passage of time and future medical historians will regard them in the same light as the convictions of medieval philosophers who argued how many angels could theoretically balance on the tip of a pin. Perhaps the next lead will come from a totally unexpected direction such as the biology of natural ageing, the recognition of some obscure environmental toxin, or some abstruse tangential spin-off of computer theory. Providing that sufficient energy, imagination, and resources are available we feel confident that the essential nature of James Parkinson's illness will eventually be disclosed.

Appendix I Some useful addresses and contacts

United Kingdom

The Parkinson's Disease Society of the United Kingdom
36 Portland Place
London W1N 3DG
Tel: 01-255-2432

The aims of this Society are to help patients and their relatives with the problems arising from Parkinson's disease, to collect and disseminate information on the illness, and to encourage and provide funds for research. There are now some thousands of active members and almost a hundred local branches. A series of helpful and practical publications are regularly produced including a newsletter. Membership is open to anyone suffering from the illness and is also open to those concerned with their welfare.

The Disabled Living Foundation
380 Harrow Road
London W9
Tel: 01-289-6111

This organization has a permanent exhibition of aids and a clothing adviser, and is a valuable source of information on equipment.

Royal Association for Disability and Rehabilitation (RADAR)
25 Mortimer Street
London W1N 8AB
Tel: 01-637-5400

This is essentially a co-ordinating body for all organizations involved with the rehabilitation and welfare of the disabled. They publish a useful book entitled *Holidays for the Physically Handicapped* (£1.30 inc. postage).

Disabled Income Group
Mill-Mead Business Centre
Mill-Mead Road
London N17
Tel: 01-801-8013

The Group runs a confidential service on a range of financial benefits, aids, and services, and publishes a book *An ABC of services and information for disabled people* (Price £1.11 inc. postage).

Scottish Information Service for the Disabled
18/19 Claremont Crescent
Edinburgh EH7 4QD
Tel: 031-556-3882

Winged Fellowship Trust Holidays for the Disabled
Angel House
Pentonville Road
London N1 9XD
Tel: 01-833-2594

Information Service for Disabled People
Northern Ireland Committee for the Handicapped
2 Annadole Avenue
Belfast BT7 3JH
Tel: 0232 640011

Gardens for the Disabled Trust
Headcorn Manor, Headcorn
Kent

SPOD (Sexual Problems of the Disabled)

An adviser is available to answer specific questions related to sexual difficulties stemming from physical disability.

49 Victoria Street
London SW1

Local Authority Social Services and Citizens Advice Bureaux

The address of your local offices will be available in Post Offices and Public Libraries.

Fitness to drive, licence, and insurance

The Department of Transport's pamphlet D100 entitled 'Driving in the United Kingdom and Abroad' obtainable from your Post Office gives important notes on driving licences. In the section devoted to physical and mental fitness it clearly states that the law requires that patients with Parkinson's disease must inform the Licensing Centre as soon as the diagnosis is made even if disabilities are mild. Your motor vehicle insurance company should also be notified at this stage; insurers may require a medical certificate of fitness to drive.

It must be stressed that many patients after commencing treatment are so much better that no difficulty arises concerning their fitness to drive and the majority of mildly affected patients encounter no difficulty with the law or insurance companies. If disabilities are severe, almost all patients sensibly give up driving of their own accord; others decide that the side-effects of their medicines such as drowsiness or dyskinesias preclude safe driving and act accordingly. Nevertheless, if you do hold a current driving licence and have not yet notified the Licensing Authority of your disability, you are advised to do so by letter addressed to:

Department of Transport
Driving and Vehicle Licensing Centre
Longview Road
Swansea SA6 7JL

A form will then be sent to you asking for further medical details about yourself and requesting permission to approach your doctors for further information. The Authority's medical adviser will then seek confidential reports of your medical condition and these are then considered on their merits in relation to the standards set out by the Medical Commission on Accident Prevention. Further reports may also be required from your hospital specialist, and an assessment by the medical officer for the Authority may also be necessary in difficult cases. The Licensing Authority then notifies you of their decision. Sometimes a fresh licence is issued for two or three years subject to review, but often your current licence will remain in force without change. If it is decided to revoke your licence or reduce its terms of validity you will be notified of how you can appeal. Organizations that can provide helpful information and advice include:

Disabled Drivers' Association, Ashwellthorpe, Norwich NR16 LEX

Disabled Drivers' Motor Club, 39 Templewood, Ealing W5. Tel: 01 998 1228

The Parkinson's Disease Society can also supply a list of sympathetic insurance companies.

Telephone amplifiers

These can be obtained from the Post Office.

America

American Parkinson Disease Association
116 John Street
New York, NY 10038

Parkinson's Disease Foundation
William Black Medical Research Building
650 West 168th Street
New York, NY 10032

United Parkinson Foundation
220 South State Street
Chicago, IL 60604

National Parkinson Foundation
1501 NW 9th Avenue
Miami FL 33136

Parkinson Association of the Rockies
1420 Ogden Street
Denver, CO 80218

Parkinsonian Society of Greater Washington
11376 Cherry Hill Rd, 204
Beltsville, MD 20705

Central Ohio Parkinson Society
3166 Redding Road
Columbus, OH 43221

Parkinson's Disease Information and Referral Center
660 S. Euclid
Box 8111
St Louis, MO 63110

Australia

Mrs M. Jackson
4 Kensington Avenue
Dianella-6062
West Australia

Parkinson's Syndrome Society
Roy Goodall
PO Box 2408
North Parramatta
New South Wales 2151

Society of Parkinson's Syndrome
Sue Focken
150 Young St
Parkside-5063
South Australia

Parkinson's Association
Roy Hemming
Tasmania
2 Kallatie Rd
Montagu Bay
Hobart
Tasmania
Australia 7018

Parkinson's Association of Western Australia
The Secretary Unit 5
85 Rokeby Road
Subiaco
Western Australia 6008
Tel: (09) 381 8699

Parkinson's Disease Association
Jim Mason
269 Auburn Road
Hawthorn
Victoria 3122

Austria

Osterreichische Parkinson Gesellschaft
POB 100
A-197 Wien
Osterreich

Belgium

Association Pour La Lutte Contre La Maladie de Parkinson, ASBL
Vereniging Voor de Strijd Tegen de Ziekte van Parkinson VZWD
Institut de Medecine
Hospital de Bavière
Bd de la Constitution 66
4000 Liege

Association Parkinson Belge
Belgische Parkinson Vereniging
c/o Paul Mengal
Rue de Culot
50-B 5991 Tourinnes-la-Grosse

Brazil

Associagao Brasil Parkinson
Marylandes Grossman
President Rua José Maria Lisbon 1.035
Apt 112 CEP 01423
Sao Paulo

Canada

Parkinson's Disease Society
1284 Clyde Avenue
Ottawa
Ontario K2C 1Y5

Parkinson Disease Foundation of Canada
Manulife Centre, Suite 232
55 Bloor Street West
Toronto
Ontario M4W 1A6

British Columbia Parkinson's Disease Association
645 West Broadway
Vancouver
British Columbia V5Z 1G6

Parkinson's Society
Beverly Boren
Suite 101
10611-84 Avenue
Edmonton
Alberta T6E 2H7

The Parkinson's Society of Alberta
10649 Suskatchewan Drive
Edmonton
Alberta T6E 4S3

Neurological Center
David Kabool
MSW 1195 W. 8th Avenue
Vancouver
British Columbia V6H 1C5

Parkinson's Disease Society
of Nova Scotia—Victor C. Johnson
PO Box 242
Station M
Halifax NS. B3J 2N7

London Parkinson
Support Group
Patrick Hailstone
363 Wortley Rd
London
Ontario N6C 3S3

Parkinson Foundation of Canada
Mr G. R. Bjornson (Montreal Chap)
Bureau 911
1155 Avenue Metculfe
Montreal
Quebec H3B 2O9

Denmark

Dansk Parkinsonforening
Lise Hoffmeyer
Tingskiftevej 8
2900 Hellerup

Eire

Information Service for the Disabled
Union of Voluntary Organisations for the Handicapped
29 Eaton Square
Monkstown
Co. Dublin

France

France Parkinson
49 rue Mirabeau
75016 Paris

L'association des Groupments de Parkinsoniens
3 Chemin du Grand Fossé-Dissignac
44600 Saint-Nazaire

Germany

Deutsche Parkinson Vereinigung e.v. Bundesverband (DPV)
Huttenstrasse 7
4040 Neuss

Hungary

Professor Eudue Csanda
Ideggdgyuszahi Kliuika
Semmelweisz University
Budapest

Israel

Mr Mordechai Yeshyrun
58376 Holon
72 Weizman Street
POB 9262
Tel-Aviv 61091

Italy

Dr Tommaso Caraceni
1st Neurologico 'C. Besta'
Via Celoria 11
20133 Milano

Japan

Tokyo Parkinson Patient's Association,
Abe Sueo,
3–12 Tsurumki 2-Chome,
Setagayaku,
Tokyo

Japan Parkinson's Association
Satoshi Fujii
979-227 Misawa
Hino-shi
Tokyo 191

Mexico

Mr Numa Usi
Paseo DeLa Soladad #86
La Herradura 53920

Netherlands

Parkinson Patienten Vereniging
Mr C. Schamhart
Postbus 46
3980 CA Bunnik

New Zealand

Mrs E. Kelly
Field Officer
Southland Parkinson's Disease Society Inc.
PO Box 1561
Invercargill

Mr H. M. Schellekena
Parkinson's Disease Society
c/o 148 England Street
Christchurch

Parkinson's Society of New Zealand
PO Box 10138
Wellington

Spain

Associació Catalana per al Parkinson
Mª A. Margarit de Sansalvador
Pau Claris 180–182. 4.° 11ª
08037 Barcelona

Parkinson Espana
Asociacion Espanola Para El Parkinson
Valencia. 304ent.2ª
08009 Barcelona

South Africa

The Secretary
South African Parkinsonian Association
CNA Building
39 Gale Street
Durban
PO Box 18151

Sweden

MS-forbundet
Riksorganisation for neurologiskt sjuka och handicappade
David Bagares gata 3
111 38 Stockholm

Staffan Wellen
Neurologiskt Handikappade
Riksforbund-Kansli:
Kungsgatan 32
111 35 Stockholm

Switzerland

Schweizerische Parkinsonvereinigung
Postfach 8128
Hinteregg

Appendix II Some helpful publications

Communication in Parkinson's Disease
Sheila Scott, F. I. Caird, and B. O. Williams
Croom Helm (1985) £7.95

Compass: The Direction Finder for Disabled People
edited by Jean MacQueen
DIG (3rd edn) (1984) £2.25

Directory for Disabled People
Ann Darnbrough and Derek Kinrade
Woodhead-Faulkner (4th edn) (1985) £17.50

Disability Rights Handbook: A guide to rights, benefits and services for all people with disabilities and their families
The Disability Alliance (published annually) (1989/90) £3.75

Door-to-Door: A guide to transport for disabled people
Department of Transport £2.50

Handicapped at Home
Sydney Foot
Design Centre Books (in association with DLF) (1977) £3.50

Help for Handicapped People
DHSS leaflet HB1 Free

Holidays in the British Isles for Disabled People
RADAR (1989) £3.00

Holidays Abroad for Disabled People
RADAR (1989) £3.00

Kitchen Sense for Disabled People of all Ages
Heinemann (in association with DLF) (1975) £9.95

Living with Parkinson's Disease
Sue Franklyn, Alison Perry, and Alison Beattie
PDS (1982) £1.00

Parkinson's: A Patient's View
Sidney Dorros
Seven Locks Press, USA (1981)

Parkinson's Disease: A guide for the patient and his family
R. C. Duvoisin
Raven Press, USA

The Parkinson's Disease Handbook
Richard Godwin-Austen
Sheldon Press

A glossary of terms

acetylcholine: the chemical messenger (neurotransmitter) released by cholinergic nerves.

adjuvant: a medicine which is added to the prescription to aid the main ingredient.

adrenalin: a hormone of the adrenal gland.

agonist: a chemical or drug that enhances neurotransmitter activity.

akinesia: marked slowness or absence of body movements.

alkaloid: a naturally occurring substance containing nitrogen which behaves chemically like an alkali, possessing important poisonous and medicinal properties.

Alzheimer's disease: a degenerative brain disorder which usually begins in middle or late adult life causing deterioration of mental abilities.

amino acids: organic compounds containing carbon, hydrogen, oxygen, and nitrogen atoms, which are the basic elements of proteins. There are about 25 in the human body. Some of these cannot be synthesized by the body and must be present in the diet.

amantadine (Symmetrel): a drug which causes an increase in dopamine release in the animal brain.

amorphous: without a fixed or regular shape.

antagonist: a substance that diminishes neurotransmitter activity.

anticholinergic: a substance which opposes the naturally occurring chemical messenger called acetylcholine.

auto-antibodies: proteins produced by the body which react with and may damage parts of the body leading to illness.

axon: a long filament of nervous tissues which conducts nervous impulses to other parts of the nervous system.

basal ganglia or nuclei: the large grey masses in the basement of the brain, concerned with the programming of normal movement.

bradykinesia: slowness in initiating and executing movements and difficulty in performing repetitive movements.

brain-stem: the lowest part of the brain connecting the cerebrum with the spinal cord.

carbidopa: a chemical which prevents the breakdown of levodopa in the body before it reaches the brain.

cerebellum: an extension of the brain-stem particularly concerned with the co-ordination of complicated movements.

cerebrum: the forebrain consisting of two large hemispheres each with its own specific function.

central nervous system: consists of the brain and spinal cord which control movement, consciousness, and mental activities.

chorea (Greek = dance): abnormal, jerky, rapid involuntary movements of the body. These occur in certain diseases such as Huntington's chorea and are also caused by excessive amounts of levodopa.

corpus striatum: a striped structure in the brain which is part of basal nuclei and is formed by two grey masses called the putamen and caudate nucleus.

decarboxylase inhibitor: a drug which blocks the action of an enzyme which converts levodopa to dopamine.

dendrite: fine branching projection of a nerve cell which receives impulses from the axons of other cells.

deprenyl: a drug which inhibits the enzyme which destroys dopamine.

disorientation: a disturbance of awareness of one's whereabouts.

dopamine: a chemical messenger derived from levodopa which is deficient in Parkinson's disease.

double-blind study: when neither the patient nor the physician knows who is receiving active medication or placebo.

dysfunction: a disorder of normal bodily activities.

dyskinesia: an involuntary and abnormal movement.

dystonia: slow, twisting, or writhing involuntary movements.

encephalitis: an inflammation of the brain usually caused by a viral infection.

encephalitis lethargica: a type of encephalitis which occurred in epidemics during 1916–26 and caused sleepiness and abnormal movements and, later, an unusual form of Parkinson's disease.

epidemiology: the study of the frequency and distribution of disease within a population.

festination: rapid, shuffling short steps when walking.

flexion: a bent, curved posture, the opposite of extension.

glaucoma: an eye disease caused by increased pressure within the eyeball.

genetic susceptibility: an inherited vulnerability to a particular disease.

haemophilia: an inherited disorder leading to spontaneous bleeding and bruising caused by a deficiency in one of the factors required for normal clotting of blood.

idiopathic: denotes a disease of unknown cause.

intercurrent infection: one which occurs in the course of another illness.

labile mood: unstable and unpredictable swings of emotion and behaviour.

leguminous: belonging to the bean or pulse family.

levodopa (L-dopa): the abbreviated chemical name of the amino acid L 3-4-dihydroxyphenylalanine.

lobe: a demarcated segment of the brain. Each cerebral hemisphere has four lobes called the frontal, temporal, parietal, and occipital.

micrographia: small handwriting which often develops in Parkinson's disease.

neural: relating to nervous tissue.

neuroleptic drug: drugs which act as dopamine antagonists and aggravate or cause the symptoms of parkinsonism.

neuron: a nerve cell.

neurotransmitter: A chemical messenger used to convey nervous messages to parts of the body.

on–off phenomenon: term used to describe abrupt and often unpredictable changes in mobility of patients with Parkinson's disease.

palaeontology: the branch of geology concerned with the study of fossil remains.

paralysis agitans: the Latin form of the older, popular term, 'shaking palsy'.

placebo: an inactive preparation resembling an active medication given to half the participants in a controlled double-blind drug trial.

psychedelic: hallucinatory or illusory effects of certain drugs.

receptor: a chemical substance fastened to the surface of a cell which responds selectively to a particular neurotransmitter.

refractory: resistant to treatment.

retardation: a slowing down of bodily or mental processes.

rigidity: a type of muscular stiffness recognized as a constant, even resistance to passive movement.

schizophrenia: a mental illness causing disintegration of the personality and producing delusions and hallucinations.

serendipity: an accidental discovery.

'shaking palsy': an old term used by James Parkinson in his original description.

sleeping sickness: popular term for encephalitis lethargica.

stereotactic surgery: an extremely accurate surgical technique for operating within the brain through a small hole in the skull.

substantia nigra: a narrow band of darkly pigmented nervous tissue in the brain-stem.

synapse: the junction between two nerve cells which is crossed by chemical messengers.

synergism: the phenomenon whereby two drugs work together so that the total effect is greater than the sum of the effects.

thalamus: a larger relay station for nerve fibres carrying sensory information situated close to the corpus striatum.

thalamotomy: the surgical procedure of accurately placing a small lesion in the thalamus.

tremor: an involuntary rhythmical oscillating movement which may affect the limbs, hand, or trunk and which commonly occurs in Parkinson's disease.

tyrosine: an amino acid occurring in nature which is the normal precursor of dopamine and adrenalin.

vesicatory: an irritant medication which when applied to the skin causes blisters to develop.

Index

acetylcholine 33–5, 61, 80
aids to daily living 58–9
amantidine (Symmetrel) 46–7, 80
America, useful addresses 69–70
anticholinergic drugs 32–5, 57–8, 80
antidepressant drugs 27, 43
anxiety 27–8
apomorphine 48, 50–1
Australia, useful addresses 70–1
Austria, useful addresses 71
auto-antibodies 29, 80
axons 7–8, 80

basal ganglia 5–6, 11–12, 80
bathing aids 59
bed, turning in 56
Belgium, useful addresses 71
benapryzine (Brizin) 33
benserazide 39, 44
benzhexol (Artane) 33, 57
benztropine (Cogentin) 33
biperiden (Akineton) 33
bladder problems 58
blood-pressure 43
bradykinesia 1, 11–12, 17–19, 81
brain implant surgery 64
brain-stem 4, 81
brain tumour 3, 6
Brazil, useful addresses 71
breathing exercises 54
bromocriptine (Parlodel) 47–8

Canada, useful addresses 72–3
carbidopa 39, 44, 81
carbon disulphide poisoning 25
carbon monoxide poisoning 25
cerebellum 4–5, 11, 81
cerebrum 4, 11, 81
chairs
    choosing 59
    rising from 14, 55
chorea 81

Citizens Advice Bureaux 67
cogwheel rigidity 17
confusion 19, 35, 44
constipation 53, 57
corpus striatum 5, 9, 11–12, 81
corticobasal degeneration 3
cramps, muscle 45–6

decarboxylase inhibitors 39, 44, 81
dendrites 7–8, 81
Denmark, useful addresses 73
deprenyl 22, 48–9, 63, 81
depression 28, 44
diet
    causing disease 25–6
    recommendations 52–3, 57
diffuse cortical Lewy body disease 3
Disabled Drivers' Association 69
Disabled Drivers' Motor Club 69
Disabled Income Group 67
Disabled Living Foundation 58, 66
disorientation 19, 81
domperidone 42
dopa 37
dopa-decarboxylase 39
dopamine 9–12, 36–7, 61, 81
    connection with Parkinson's disease
      9–11
    deficiency 11–12
    effects on mood 11, 28
    functions 10–11
    interactions with acetylcholine 33–4
dopamine agonists 48, 50
dressing 14, 58
dribbling of saliva 18–19, 57
drive, fitness to 68–9
drug holidays 50
drug-induced parkinsonism 3, 10,
      26–7, 34
dyskinesias 81
    interdose 45
    L-dopa-induced 45, 62–3
    tardive 27

eating aids 58–9
Eire, useful addresses 73
Eldepryl, *see* deprenyl
emotional stress 15–16, 27–8
encephalitis lethargica 23–4, 81–2
exercises 53–6

facial appearance 13–14
fainting 43
festination 82
France, useful addresses 74
freezing attacks 18, 49–50, 62
  overcoming 54–6

gait, *see* walking
gamma-aminobutyric acid 61
Gardens for the Disabled Trust 67
genetic susceptibility 22–3, 65, 82
Germany, useful addresses 74
glaucoma 35, 82
globus pallidus 5

hallucinations 44, 48
handwriting 14, 41
head injury 28–9
Hungary, useful addresses 74
hydrocephalus 3

Information Service for Disabled People
  67
inheritance 22–3, 65
insomnia 57–8
intellect 19–20
Israel, useful addresses 74
Italy, useful addresses 74

Jakob-Creuzfeldt disease 63–4
Japan, useful addresses 75

Kuru 63–4

laxatives 57
levodopa (L-dopa) 10, 34, 36–46, 82
  benefits 40–2
  interactions with other drugs 43–4
  on-off effects, *see* on-off phenomenon
  proprietary preparations 39–40
  reasons for delayed action 38–9
  side-effects 42–6, 62–3
Lewy bodies 7
libido 44, 58
lisuride 48, 50

Madopar 39–40
magnetic resonance imaging (MRI)
  60–1
manganese miners 25
memory 19
mental changes 19–20, 44
mercury poisoning 25
methixene (Tremonil) 33
methyl alcohol poisoning 25
Mexico, useful addresses 75
micrographia 82
monoamine oxidase inhibitors 43, 48–9
mood, effects of dopamine 11, 28
movement
  disorders, *see* bradykinesia; dyskinesias;
    tremor
  influence of dopamine 10–11
  nervous system control 4–6
MPTP 22, 27
muscle stiffness, *see* rigidity
music therapy 54

nerve cells (neurons) 7–9
nervous system 3–6
Netherlands, useful addresses 75
neuropeptides 61
neurotransmitters 8–9, 61, 82
  see also acetylcholine *and* dopamine
New Zealand, useful addresses 75–6

occupational therapists 58
oculogyric crisis 24
on-off phenomenon 42, 49, 82
  management 50–1, 53, 62
orphenadrine (Disipal) 33, 57

paralysis agitans 83
Parkinson, James 1–2
Parkinson's Disease Society of the United
  Kingdom 58, 66
Parkinson's syndromes 3
personality 19, 28
physical activity 53–6
physiotherapy 50, 54

placebo effect 31
poisons, environmental 25
positron emission tomography (PET) 61
post-encephalitic parkinsonism 24–5, 34
posture 18, 19
   correcting 54, 56
potassium cyanide poisoning 25
procyclidine (Kemadrin) 33
punch-drunk boxers 28
pyridoxine 43–4

Rauwolfia serpentina 9–10
reflex movements 5
relaxation techniques 54
reserpine 10
rigidity 1, 12, 16–17, 83
   cogwheel 17
Royal Association for Disability and Rehabilitation (RADAR) 66

saliva, dribbling 18–19, 57
Scottish Information Service for the Disabled 67
scrapie 63
selegiline, see deprenyl
sensory reinforcement 54
sexual difficulties 58
Sexual Problems of the Disabled (SPOD) 67
shaking palsy 2, 83
Sinemet 39–40
smoking, cigarette 3
Social Services, Local Authority 58, 67
South Africa, useful addresses 76
Spain, useful addresses, 76
spasms, muscle 45–6
speech
   exercises 56
   problems 18
spinal cord 4–5
Steele-Richardson-Olszewski syndrome 3

stereotactic surgery 16, 36, 83
stress, emotional 15–16, 27–8
strio-nigral degeneration 3
strokes 3
substantia nigra 5, 9, 11–12, 83
   fetal implants 64
   post-mortem abnormalities 6–7
surgical treatments 16, 35–6, 64
Sweden, useful addresses 76
Switzerland, useful addresses 77
synapses 8–9, 83

tardive dyskinesia 27
telephone amplifiers 56, 69
thalamus 5, 12, 83
toxins, environmental 25
tranquillizers
   major 26–7, 44
   minor 27, 43
Transport, Department of 68
tremor 1, 12, 15–16, 83
   essential 22
tyrosine 37–8, 83

United Kingdom, useful addresses 66–9

vibration treatment 32
virus infections 23–5
vitamin B6 43–4
vomiting 11, 42–3

walking 14–15, 18–19
   aids 59
   recommendations 53–5
weight control 52–3
Wilson's disease 3
Winged Fellowship Trust Holidays for the Disabled 67